THE SECRETS OF
MUSICALITY
FOR DANCERS

LEARNING 9 ESSENTIAL
MUSICALITY SKILLS
IN DANCE

KRISTOFER MENCÁK

ONLINE:
musicalitycourse.com
youtube.com/@kristofermencak
facebook.com/kristofermencakdancer
instagram.com/kizombaflow
tiktok.com/kristofermencak

kizombaclasses.com

ISBN: 9798676799410
Imprint: Independently published

OTHER BOOKS BY KRISTOFER MENCÁK

In the Dance Series

"The Secrets of Social Dance – How to Become a Popular Dancer", on Amazon.com.

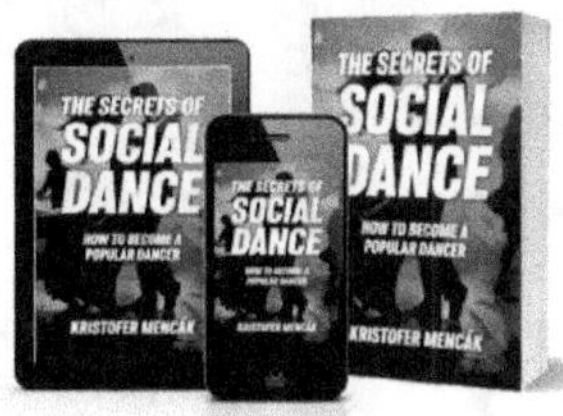

Other

"Unsuck Life – The tips tools & trick for how to change what sucks and improve what doesn't", on Amazon.com.

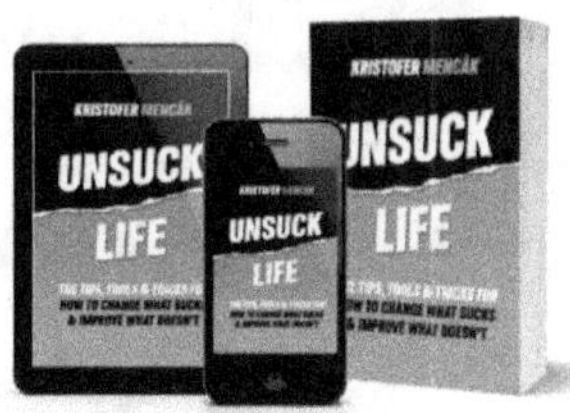

TABLE OF CONTENTS

PREFACE

Never in my life I expected to do this. Write a book about musicality. To be honest, I never even expected to become a dance teacher. But for the last six years it has been my full-time job. I have travelled to more than 150 cities in more than 60 countries all over the world. I have visited some places I never expected to visit, many places more than once and some places several times per year.

Like I mentioned, I am a dance teacher. I am not a musician. But I love music. And my dancer's perspective on musicality and how to teach it for dancers has become incredibly popular. I am happy to have helped so many people learn how to listen to music and play with it on the dance floor. And this is also why I decided to write this book, to share it with as many people as possible.

It all started out from elaborating on the notes I had for my own musicality classes, and then it has gradually expanded. I have learned a lot just putting words to my thoughts but also from trying to research as much as I can about music and musicality for dance.

My hope is that you will learn a lot too, that it will open your ears to the music. Because dancing with the music is so much better than just taking steps or making moves without any connection to it.

Just like my previous book, *Unsuck Life*, I will try to be brief and to the point. I want you to get as much value as possible from each chapter and paragraph in this book, so I try to keep most of the fluff out, but there are some repetitions, I admit.

HOW TO READ THIS BOOK

First of all, I have tried to write this book for any kind of dancer - solo dancers and couple dancers alike. Even if there are many different elements in music, and each genre has its own peculiarities, I believe the tools we can use to play with the music and show it in our dance are the same for all of them.

No matter if you are a hip-hop dancer or a ballet dancer, if you dance tango, dancehall, lindy hop, Latin dances or kizomba my hope is that you will find a lot of new insights and ideas in this book. Sometimes it might be old news, sometimes it might be totally new and sometimes it might be something you knew but didn't really have the words to describe or the tools to put in your dance.

There are many different skills in musicality. In this book I will try to cover all that I currently teach in my live workshops as well as some things that I rarely have time for.

If you really want to get better musicality and get the most out of the book there is also a course with more than 60 exercises, several for each chapter. You can find it all online when you go to www.musicalitycourse.com. This book and the musicality course there go hand in hand.

The first part of the book is an introduction to music and musicality, what it is, why it is needed, and why it is sometimes missing.

The second part is also short and more theoretical, about music theory. How music is built. A musician doesn't need to know anything about dance unless they want to make music that is great for dancing. But a dancer has a lot to gain from knowing a bit about music, since we normally dance to music in one form or another. If you are a teacher, it is great to know this and be able to explain it in class. But learning music theory is not the main purpose of this book, so we don't go into much detail.

If you don't really care about this second part, or already know, you can skip ahead and go straight to the third part of the book. But some things might be easier to understand if you have read the second part.

The third part of the book is about the connection between musicality and dance, and why it is so important with this connection.

The fourth part is the bulk of this book. This is where we will really try to break it down and figure out what we can listen to, how we can play with the music - in short, how we can improve our musicality. We will look at different skills in musicality and how to use them.

If you are a musician, please sit down and practice deep nasal breathing while reading. This is a book aimed at dancers, and some terminology is not the same as for a musician. Some terminology is also used in different ways. I don't want you to suffer a heart attack. Relax.

Reading through this book, we will get better at understanding exactly how we can listen more to the music and express it better in our dancing. But we will only get better on one condition. Only if we practice. Only if we dance. A lot.

Now let's get to it!

PART ONE - INTRODUCTION

What is Musicality?

Within the dancing world, we use the word "musicality". We try to be "musical", but what does it really mean? We have some kind of idea. We talk about it. There are classes on it. And quite often we know it when we see it. But can we explain it? If I would ask you what musicality is, how would you define it? And would others define it in the same way?

I think there would be a lot of different answers. Some would simply talk about "understanding the music", but I think that is both too vague and too limited.

To vague, because what does that really mean? Understanding the music?

And too limited because I think musicality is more than that. It is not something purely intellectual, like "understanding". Musicality has an expressive side too. I think it isn't just one thing. It has many different layers or skills. It is not that easy to define, but we will give it a try.

But before we dive into that, let's first take a glance at what music is. Quite often it is contrasted with noise and randomness. Noise is not very pleasant, so music should hopefully be pleasant to listen to. And since it is contrasted with randomness, music should also be deliberate and planned in some way. There should be some thought behind it. Some kind of idea behind the sounds that we hear when we listen to music. This is good to have in mind when we talk about it. And we will come back to it later.

Returning to musicality, it can be different things for different people. There is no clear definition accepted by all, and even though many people say they want better musicality, what they mean by it might differ, since musicality is also something personal. We like different music, and our way of hearing and expressing music is also different.

Musicality is personal, but if we want to improve it, we need to start from somewhere. We need to have a starting point, some kind common understanding of what it is so that we can figure out how we can improve it.

The definition we will use in this book is from Wikipedia:

> *"A person considered musical has the ability to perceive and reproduce differences in aspects of music including pitch, rhythm, and harmony. Two types of musicality may be differentiated: to be able to perceive music (musical receptivity) and to be able to reproduce music in addition to creating music (musical creativity)."*

Now we have something to work with. For a dancer, the exact definition of musicality can be similar, but not exactly the same.

The ability to perceive music would still be the same. How good are we at noticing what is happening in the music? How well do we hear the different aspects of music?

The second part would be a bit different though. We neither reproduce nor create music. We would still need to be able to express different aspects of music, but we are dancers. We create dance. Our instrument is our body, or bodies in the case of couple dancing.

So, a dancer would need to be able to perceive differences in aspects of music, interpret them in a creative way and then also express these differences in the dance. These are the core elements of musicality for dancers.

If I make a more personal interpretation I would say that the creativity for a dancer can be expressed as an ability to connect with the music and interpret it, making movements that relate to the music in a way that makes sense, both visually and in how they feel in the body. In a way it should be possible to "see the music" when we see dance. Even if we would turn the music off, the moves should still look like the music sounds. Does that make sense?

And a move should "feel right in the body". In a way it should feel as the sound sounds. Or maybe the move should look like it could produce that sound. There needs to be a connection between the sound and the move. They should work together.

So, to be musical we have to be able to perceive the music. And we also have to be creative in how we interpret it and express it. Only one of those skills is not enough. We need it all. Just perceiving the music doesn't help us expressing it in a creative way. And just being able to express it doesn't help that much if we can't perceive all the nuances in the music. And we need to be creative to connect the music with the dance in a good way.

A Metaphor

Now I would like to introduce a metaphor here, something that we will return to over and over, and which will hopefully make it easier to understand.

I would like to think of music as one language (the source language) that we have to translate into another language – dance (the target language). I am the dancer and therefore I am the translator, but none of the languages is my mother tongue. The better I can perceive the music, the better my understanding of the source language. If I don't perceive music very well, I will not be able to translate it very well either.

And if I want to translate the music into dance in a good way, I also need to know the target language, dance. A translator needs to know both languages well. The worse my dance skills, the more limited my expression will be. If I don't have very good technique, or I don't have that many moves, it is the same as having bad pronunciation or a limited vocabulary. It will be difficult to express myself well. The dance might be a bit stiff, maybe not very varied.

But even if we know both languages, it doesn't necessarily mean we will be good translators. It doesn't mean we will be musical. We might lack some skills that a translator need. Maybe we will not find the right words, or we don't find them fast enough. Maybe we will not find the right nuances. Maybe we can't translate the right feeling.

For dancers, if we are missing the creative part of musicality, we might not be very good translators of the music.

We might perceive the music well, and we might have a good "vocabulary" in dance, but we still don't find the right word. We will still miss the feeling of the dance.

The better we are, the more our dance will match the source language, the music, and the richer the translation will be.

So, we have found something to work with. We know we need to improve how we perceive music. We know we have to listen to different aspects of music. And we know we have to become creative in how we express what we hear when we dance.

So, for example, musicality can be how we can catch many different aspects in a song and represent them with our bodies. It is dancing to the rhythm. It is changing tempos and the timing of moves to fit with the music. It is catching the dominant feeling of a song. It is catching different aspects of specific sounds, whether it is the size of the moves, the level we make the move on, or how soft it is. It is using silence in music. It is predicting the music, what is going to happen, and preparing for what to do with it. It is using the vocals, sometimes playing with different words and actions in the music. And it is even using breathing in our dance, in a way that also plays with the music. And finally, what really sets a dancer apart, it is picking and choosing from all of the above, combining this into a whole, expressing the music through the body.

Musicality is dancing not just to one instrument, but to several different instruments, all the time picking and choosing which sound we want to highlight, and sometimes even dancing to several instruments at the same time.

Musicality is one of the signs of a more advanced dancer - someone who is able to hear what the music calls for and express it in dance. When we become better dancers, we listen more to the music. And when we listen more to the music, we become even better dancers.

Two Different Ways to Express Musicality

Musicality can be expressed in two very distinct ways. One is through choreography, often on a stage. For a choreography the choreographer had time to listen to the music many many times and was able to decide exactly what move to do at each point in time, to each sound they wanted to express. Performing choreography is like dancing with a script. We know beforehand exactly what to do, when to do it and how to do it. How well it fits the music depends on the musicality of the choreographer, and a little bit on how the dancer interprets the moves he or she is instructed to do.

Another way to express musicality is on the dance floor. In a way, this is like jazz music. It is totally improvised. At each moment in time, we have to decide what sound to express and how to express it. Maybe we can demand more musicality from a choreography, since a choreographer has time to plan each and every move, really adapting it to the music. But I believe dancing on the social floor puts more pressure on the dancer. On the floor the dance has to be created on the fly, "choreographed" all while we dance, maybe even during the very first time we hear that song. This also means that no dance will be exactly the same on the social floor. Every dance, with each and every partner, will be unique.

The way we use our musicality in these cases can be different. But we need both the receptive and the creative skills for both choreography and on the dance floor. The only real difference is how much time there is to create the dance.

Why Musicality is Lacking?

I believe that there is a lack of musicality on many dance floors, at least within the dance subculture I come from. I see a couple of different reasons for this. One of the most important of those are us, the teachers.

The Teacher's Role

When a student wants to learn more about musicality, it is pretty natural that they seek out more classes about musicality.

But from my own experience, it can be difficult to find good classes. Musicality is often not the focus in regular classes. Many regular classes emphasize steps and moves.

If we think of our translation metaphor, it is like most classes are focused only on the target language. As if a non-native English to Spanish translator only tried to learn Spanish. It wouldn't be the greatest translations ever made without knowing English well.

I cannot say exactly what kind of regular classes are given where you live. It all differs from school to school, city to city, and country to country. There are many good teachers and also many not so good teachers. You might have been lucky. But like I mentioned, I haven't experienced many, if any, pure musicality classes when I have taken regular classes myself.

To be perfectly honest, when I was new in teaching, I didn't really teach much musicality in my own regular classes either. I was too amazed by steps and moves myself. And then I quit giving regular classes to focus only on traveling and teaching. So, I didn't do a good job in my own town. I believe I have done a better job teaching musicality during the more recent years in workshops and festivals all over the world. This brings me to the second type of class.

In dance festivals, I would guess only around 5-10 % of classes are dedicated to music or musicality. Since most regular and festival classes are dedicated to steps or moves it creates the impression that this is what is most important to become a good dancer. Yes, all people who are learning how to dance need to learn how to move, the specifics for that dance, but it is not all they need to learn. And I don't think 5-10 % is the right proportion. Such a low percentage doesn't send the right signal of just how important musicality really is for a dancer.

Another problem is that the musicality classes in festivals often come in two different kinds.

Choreography Class

Either the musicality class is really more about choreography. A dance teacher has chosen a piece of a song he or she likes, has decided on a certain sequence of steps, with a certain timing that in their opinion fits the chosen music well. And then in class, the students learn that choreography to that part of the song. Yes, there might be some value to this approach, if the teacher explains what he or she is listening to in the music, why they chose to dance to certain sounds and why they chose to express those sounds in that way.

However, there is one big problem with this type of class. It is still just the teacher's interpretation of the music. It is not the student's interpretation. If we go back and look at the definition of musicality, it is not the students that learn how to perceive the music and practice their creativity in expressing it.

If we return to our metaphor, it is as if the teacher gave the student a new sentence in Spanish:

"One beer, please. = Una cerveza, por favor."

However useful that phrase might be, it still covers quite a small part of the Spanish language. Maybe someday in the future we will want to say something else? Maybe we want to understand when we can use certain words and how we can combine them in the best way possible.

Returning to teaching musicality, another disadvantage is the fact that the students might not hear that song on the dance floor for a week or a month or longer. And when they finally do, they might not remember what they were supposed to do. But once again, it is still not their musicality. So, the only real value would be in the explanations the teacher gave in class - why they are dancing in a certain way to a certain part of the music or a specific sound. And it is not always that this is explained.

Theoretical Class

Another type of musicality class is a more theoretical class which is really more about how the musicians create that kind of music, the different instruments used, the functions of those instruments, the normal rhythms of those instruments in that type of music, the structure of that type of music and maybe how to distinguish between different types of music that is similar.

If we imagine our translation metaphor again, it is like a class about spelling rules in the source language when what we really need is to learn to translate. We are not required to do anything with the source language anyway. It might be good to know, but we will not produce anything in the source language.

Yes, this kind of class can be important in a theoretical way, both for students and even more so for teachers. It is a theory class. But the students don't really get to practice much, if at all. They don't get to dance in different ways. And most important of all, they don't really learn how to listen to the music and express it as they hear it. So, this type of class also misses the core elements of musicality.

Musicality is Something Else

To me, neither of these is really about musicality. One is really a choreography class, where the teacher is the one showing his or her musicality and the students are learning that choreography. It is creating a carbon copy of the teacher's way of hearing the music. And the other is a kind of theory class on musical structure, instruments, or differences between different types of music. In my opinion, neither of these classes practice much on the "being receptive" part of musicality. And they don't practice at all on the "being creative" part. I believe musicality should be taught in a different way.

The Student's Role

Leaders Focus on Steps & Moves

It is not only the teachers' fault that musicality is lacking though. When we start learning how to dance, we are very focused on learning moves. Especially when we dance couple dances socially, the leaders often don't listen much to the music. The focus is on steps and moves, on trying to lead what is in our mind, on a technical level. To be fair, it is actually not that easy to lead. It requires a lot of focus. So, we dedicate ourselves to this. Practicing the moves that have been taught in class, seen on the dance floor or in some video on YouTube. Part of this focus on steps might be because there are so few musicality classes, so it is not perceived as something very important nor anything we need to practice.

In addition, leaders are constantly trying to learn new moves that we try to lead, and when learning new moves, we always need to pay attention to them. We always need to focus on the leading. And we continue learning new moves until we feel we have reached a decent level and have a good repertoire. Only then do we start to relax a bit more and have more capacity to focus on other things.

If we think about our translation metaphor, it is as if the leaders are trying to squeeze in advanced and rarely used words like circumlocution, diaphanous or legerdemain in the translation, instead of really listening to the source language. Usually it would make more sense to learn how to interpret the source language better. The same goes for musicality.

Better to focus more on the music, trying to understand it, than learning super advanced moves that are done without connection to the music.

Followers Prefer Musicality

As a beginner dancer, followers also don't have the freedom to listen to the music very much. A follower needs to focus on following, on interpreting the signals the leader is sending. All the attention goes towards that. And therefore, it is difficult to pay close attention to the music and develop much musicality.

However, I think that followers have the opportunity to start listening to the music earlier than leaders. Maybe because they often get to a decent level in following before leaders feel they have enough moves. And therefore, they have some mental capacity free and can pay more attention to the music.

One of the followers' most common complaints is that, in general, leaders listen too little to the music, and try too much to execute different moves. Therefore, my guess is that followers actually can free themselves from the focus on following earlier than leaders can stop focusing on leading.

When traveling the world teaching, I have often asked this question to followers: Do you prefer musicality, or do you prefer steps and moves? All over the world, the answer is always the same - musicality wins all the time. There might be some followers who say they like steps more, or that they want both steps and musicality, but there is always a vast majority who say they prefer to dance with a leader who listens to the music before one who has a great repertoire of steps and moves they do. This is something worth remembering for leaders who want to be appreciated on the dance floor.

Focus on Musicality

When we start dancing it is important to realize that musicality is much more important for dance than what we initially think. We should really try to spend less time thinking only about technique and moves and instead start paying more attention to the music, as early as possible. We need to better balance our skills in the source and target language. We need to practice listening to and interpreting the music just as much as we practice the technique, practice how to best express the music. We don't have to be great dancers to start paying attention to the music. We can start practicing on our creative interpretation of the music from day one when we start dancing.

Why Teach Technique?

This might seem a bit hypocritical. I teach a lot of technique too. Why do I spend so much time on technique when I say musicality is so important and valued more? Well, I still think technique is very important, for a variety of reasons. And it is important for both leaders and followers.

Good Technique Leads to Better Dancing

First of all, it makes the dance technically better. When we dance couple dances there is always leading and following. The leader sends a signal and the follower has to interpret that signal. With better technique, the leader will send a clearer signal so there will be less guessing and back-leading. And the timing of the leading will be better. The follower will be better at listening to and reacting to the signal. The interpretation will also be better. And the execution of steps or moves from the follower will be better, with better timing.

The leader then needs to listen to the feedback from the follower. Is the interpretation of the leading correct? Or was there some misunderstanding?

If the follower had good technique, there will be less problems that need to be adapted to. It might be easier to listen to the feedback. And the leader might also learn there is less need for force in the leading. The leader can be gentler.

With better technique, both partners have better balance, which makes everything easier. In solo dances, everything becomes better too. Balance is better. The execution of moves is better. Control is better. These are some of the reasons for teaching technique.

Good Technique Leads to Better Musicality

If we move on to the musicality aspect of teaching technique, with better technique everything will also fit better with the timing of the music. It is one thing to step with the same tempo as the music. But another to be on beat as opposed to slightly off beat or to vary slightly with steps that are a bit too fast or too slow relative to the beat.

Like we just mentioned, with better technique in both leading and following the signal sent and the interpretation of that signal will be better. The resulting steps will be more on time with the music, and better matching the intention from the leader. So, everything that is done will be done more synchronized with the music.

With more technique we will also have a greater repertoire of steps and moves. And we can use these to express ourselves better to the music. We have more types of moves and many moves of each type so we can fit them to the music in better ways. We will have more possibilities and better expression to the music.

When we have a really good technique, we can lead pretty much any move better to the music. If we really make the effort to listen to it. And this is important. Often we start really listening to the music only when the technique is better, when the leading and following has become pretty automatic, in muscle memory. Then a leader starts paying attention to how to lead moves *with the music* instead of just paying attention to *how* to lead them. Once we have better technique it becomes possible to speed up or down, to transform a move into a slower one, or a faster one, within the same sequence of steps.

And when the follower has a better technique it is possible to relax more, think less of what to do, and more on how to do it. With really good technique we can change how we do a move. We can give it a different feeling.

Confidence in our technique gives us the freedom to really listen to the music. Then we can better choose what to do and also how we do those moves, to adapt it even more to the music.

Teaching Musicality

Nature vs Nurture

Some people would say that it is not possible to teach musicality. It is something you are born with. They would say either you have it, or you don't.

I don't agree. If it was that simple, we would have the people who have it, and they would all be great. And we would have the ones who don't have it, and they would all suck. I don't think this is what we see. I think some people have it more and some have it less.

Some people might be more "gifted" and have a natural talent for it. We all lie somewhere along a scale when it comes to different talents. We might be talented for some things and not so talented for others.

So, nature plays a role. But we also have the fact that some have been exposed to more music and dance since very early in their life. They have practiced more.

This is the constant debate on nature vs nurture. I think in most areas of life both nature and nurture have a role. Some things we are simply born to do, and some things we need to practice a lot. Some people have already practiced their musicality, like a musician for example. They might have a head start when it comes to perceiving music. But for all of us who are not musicians, we are not doomed. There is still hope. Nurture almost always plays a role. No matter the exact percentage of nature's and nurture's influence, I think everyone can improve their musicality a lot.

Yes, I have met students who seemed to lack both musicality and body control, but that doesn't mean it was impossible to teach them. I have seen with my own eyes how they improved. They just needed some more practice.

Our brains are extremely plastic. They can change, they can adapt. And they get good at what we practice a lot. This is something I mentioned in my previous book, *Unsuck Life*.

As an example, I can tell you about something that happened to me in Brazil, during the carnival many years ago. It was warm and I was in the pool cooling down a bit. There by the poolside I saw a four-year-old girl dancing and moving in ways that would make many girls in the Northern Hemisphere jealous. But I realized there and then that this was not necessarily talent. She had been exposed to dancing and music since she was born. Maybe she heard music already in her mother's belly. She had seen her sister dance before she could even stand up. She had been surrounded by dance and music in her neighborhood and in the media. She had imitated, and over time she became good. I think it is the same with musicality.

We might start at different ages. Some start earlier, like the girl in Brazil. Some start later, like I did. And just like it is easier to learn languages when we are small, it might be easier if we start dancing or start practicing musicality when we are young. But I know for sure we can get better at both dancing and musicality, no matter the age.

Everyone has Musicality

Imagine someone who really seems to have zero musicality. Everything seems "wrong". Do you think it would be possible for this person to tell you if one song is faster or slower than another song? If you say yes, it means they must have some musicality. Do you think it would be possible to teach someone like that to tap with their hand on the table once every second, more or less? With some practice, would it be possible to teach them to be pretty accurate in tapping their hand on the table to some music playing?

I believe so and I think you too. It is definitely possible to teach musicality, and a lot of more complicated aspects of it than this. And I believe we all have musicality if we just pay attention and really listen to the music. From there it is just a lot of practice.

In my musicality workshops, there is a moment that always tells me everyone has musicality. I ask people to listen to a specific song and think about how they want to move their body to it when they dance. I ask them to focus on the body movement, not on steps or anything else. The instructions are not more detailed than that, so there is sometimes some confusion on what it is that I want them to do. But once I put the song on, everyone gets it.

Everyone is doing the same. All students move their bodies a bit more in response to that song, a bit more body movement. It tells me there are some fundamental aspects of music that we all can understand. There is something in all music that we interpret in similar ways. It is a universal language that we all have a talent for. A language that we all can learn to both understand and speak. That moment in class tells me everyone has it.

And I believe it can be taught. I think we just need to try to awaken this sensitivity to music a bit earlier, and even more than that, we need to pay more attention to music when we dance.

For this, I think we need to have more musicality classes. We need to have better musicality classes. This book is one small attempt to make it a bit better. The written word can reach further and reach more people than I can ever hope to do in my live classes. And together with the online musicality course I also offer on www.musicalitycourse.com, anyone can learn.

Be More Musical

Sometimes students are told to try to be more musical. It is not very helpful. It is like telling a football player to play better.

Another tip that might be slightly more helpful is when they are told to listen to a lot of music. I think this is actually pretty good advice. It doesn't really teach the students anything concrete, or how to listen and interpret music. But at least they will know more songs, and they will start understanding the structure of the music subconsciously. With time this makes them better at predicting what will happen in the music, even if it is the first time they hear a song. This can definitely help them on the dance floor.

Watching more football might make us better in some way, just like listening to music might help for musicality. But playing more football will help us much more, in the same way as dancing more will. And if we really want to improve, we should probably both be playing more and trying to figure out what to work on, how we can improve.

How can we learn to be more musical? Listening to more music can help a little. And dancing more will probably help even more. But what can we do to really take it to the next level?

If we want to improve on our perception, maybe we need to some tips on what is it in the music we could listen to? And for the creative side, can we get some ideas on how to express ourselves to the music? What is it that we can consciously work on now when we practice or dance socially to be more musical later without even thinking about it?

Another Way to Teach

I don't think there is a need to tell students what to do. I think they just need some tools to help them listen to the music and express it in their dance. It is not enough to say, "just feel it" or "try to listen to the music". It has to be a bit more specific. What is happening in the music? What can we listen to? And how could that be expressed in dance?

In addition to the tools, I think students just need more freedom to express themselves. The freedom to listen to the music and explore how to express it themselves, without being told what to do or given moves from their teacher.

Part of the reason they need more freedom is because musicality is not something objective. Even if I personally think there are ways to dance to a song that make more sense, everybody hears music in a slightly different way. There is a lot of room for individual interpretation. Musicality is subjective.

And someone's musicality might also change over time, from one year to another, depending on the current mood they are in and even depending on who they are dancing with.

Learning Musicality

If we for some reason think we already are musical and that we already know and express musicality we might be falling into a trap. It might be correct that we have some musicality. We might be expressing musicality on the dance floor. At least we are using the things that "we know that we know". This is what we are aware of. But there might also be things that "we don't know that we don't know". The things we are ignorant about. These are the layers of musicality that we don't yet know.

If we believe we already have it then we will not make any effort to improve. And if we don't make any effort to improve, we will never even know what we are missing out on.

Like already mentioned, I believe everyone has musicality, but I also believe no one has perfect musicality. Musicality is not science. It is not objective. It is subjective. It is something personal. And therefore, it cannot be perfect. Since no one is perfect, we have to recognize that we all can improve. Even if we might be advanced dancers, there is still always room for improvement.

Actually, anyone, independent of their level, could teach us something. Another person might hear something in the music that we don't. If they see us dance, they might be able to give us tips on how to improve, even if we think that we overall are a better dancer than they are.

I personally love watching other people dance on the social floor, even if I rarely get the chance. Because when I watch others, I get the chance to see how other people dance, how other people hear the music and choose to express it.

When we understand that no one is perfect and that anyone can teach us something we also realize we should stay humble and not look down on other dancers for "not having musicality". The same way that we have to understand there is no perfect dancer and we all can improve our dancing.

This idea that we all have musicality, but that no one has perfect musicality is important. It can give us hope. We all have it inside and can actually start working on improving it. And since there is no objectively perfect musicality, no official right and wrong, it also takes the pressure off a bit. It might make it easier to dare to express ourselves on the dance floor.

We are all on a journey to become better dancers and better at translating music into dance. We all start from somewhere. And we have all been beginners at some point.

It doesn't help to be self-conscious and fear what other people might think. When we are self-conscious, we hardly dare to try and we cannot focus enough on what we are supposed to do.

A better approach is to not care about what other people think and practice. A lot.

PART TWO - ABOUT MUSIC

The Elements of Music

Music is built on the interplay of three things:

- Rhythm
- Melody
- Harmony

Let's take a closer look at each one of these elements.

Rhythm

Rhythm is essential for music. It is the element of time in music. When we clap our hands or tap our foot to the music, we are expressing one part of rhythm, the pulse.

Just like most things in nature, like the heart, the waves on the beach or the night and day rhythm, all music has a pulse, at a specific tempo. This is the same as when we often talk about beat, and the beat of music. From now on we will use the word beat instead of pulse, as I think it is more common among dancers. The tempo of this beat is what we often call BPM (Beats Per Minute). We don't hear the beat all the time, it is not always represented in the music, but it is there. The BPM can increase or decrease, but it usually stays the same throughout a song.

Rhythm is built on this beat, but rhythm is not only a constant beat. The beat is like a framework or a skeleton on which the rhythm is built. The rhythm is how the sounds are placed in time, how they are interspersed and the duration of them, all in relation to this beat. The different sounds that create the rhythm can be placed both on this beat, but also off. And it is the different placements of notes that create the rhythm.

Melody

The melody is what makes us immediately recognize a song. It is what makes a song really unique. It is what we would normally try to sing if we want to explain to a friend what song we are thinking of.

If only the percussion or the bass line is played it can be very hard to recognize the music, but if someone sings or plays the melody we usually can. It expresses an element of time in music, with the addition of different pitches.

The melody consists of two things. We need different notes played one after another. This gives us the ups and downs of the melody. But, to create melody we also need a rhythm element. We need to have the duration of those sounds, for how long a note is played. Together, these two create the melody and make it recognizable.

Harmony

The harmony often sets the feeling of a song and is a combination of sounds. It is what is produced when more notes are played together. If the melody is how the music progresses over time, the harmony describes the music at each point in time.

Harmony can be produced with one instrument when several notes are played at the same time. Together the different notes produce chords. Harmony can also be created with several instruments, when different notes from different instruments interact.

When we talk about harmony we also often talk about consonance and dissonance. Consonance is when chords sound smooth and pretty soft. Dissonance is when it sounds harsher, and these chords create a certain tension.

The harmony can often create different feelings in us, depending on the different combinations of chords played.

Beat, Tempos, Measures & More

Music is often contrasted with noise and randomness. But that doesn't sound very flattering in itself. It is like saying that someone is "not ugly". It doesn't really tell how great music can be. It doesn't tell us anything of the emotions it can provoke. And it doesn't really define it. It just kind of says what it is not.

The opposite of randomness is predictability or consistency. For us to be able to predict something there needs to be some kind of pattern or structure we can recognize.

We already talked about the beat that usually is continuous and doesn't change over time. This beat has a certain tempo which we usually call BPM. And this beat is usually written in a series of "bars" or "measures" on a partiture with five staves.

Most modern music has a 4/4 time signature, with space for four quarter-notes (what dancers would call beats) per measure. This means that each measure only has four beats. Usually, the first one is stronger followed by three weaker ones. Within a measure there may or may not be any notes. And if there are, the notes can be half notes, quarter notes, eighth notes, rests or whatever the composer wants. The vertical placement of the notes represents the note value. And the actual type of note represents how long it sounds. However, all note and rest values within a measure must equal to the top number (or numerator) of the time signature when they are combined.

In modern music that we dance to we very often talk about the 8-count and when we do, it is two measures we are using. So, a musician would count, 1, 2, 3, 4, 1, 2, 3, 4. And a dancer would count from 1-8. For dancers (except waltz), the 8-count is fundamental to understand.

When we dance, we use the 8-count to understand the structure of music better. In a way, it gives us a sense of place. Where are we in the music right now? Are we on one, two, three, or where? A teacher might tell us when to do a move. So, it can help us also in class.

Understanding Counting in Class

There seems to be some different ways of counting within dance teaching. But I believe there is one "right" way of doing it. And this is the one which is connected to the music we hear. When we dance, and especially in class, we usually start moving on one and we prepare for the movement with a "count up" which goes 5, 6, 7, 8.

When we want to indicate something on tempo, we count 1, 2, 3, 4, 5, 6, 7, 8, matching the two measures of music that make up that 8-count.

If we want to indicate half tempo, we can count 1, 3, 5, 7. And then we extend the duration of each number to two beats. But what do we do if we want to indicate double tempo? Easy. We count and 1 and 2 and 3 and 4 and so on. Every "and" also indicates a move. These three tempos cover most of what we need on the dance floor. But it is possible to dance and count faster or slower. If we want to be even faster, we can count e and a 1 e and a 2 e and a 3 e and a 4 and so on. This way we get four moves in one beat in the music and we would indicate 32 moves within a normal 8-count. And we could also count just 1, 5 if we want to indicate something super slow. Combining all these, we get the pattern count, connecting the moves we do with the music we hear.

But it important to notice that there shouldn't be any vocalization if there is no move, especially for the "and"s. It would make no sense. Maybe the exception would be to say "hold" or something similar on a count where we don't move or make a weight transfer. But then it would make most sense to do just that - substitute the number with a word that gives some instruction that there should be no movement. Making a normal count when there is no move could be confusing.

Phrases

Different sections of the music, like intro, verses, chorus etc. are built on phrases. Together they form a structure for each song. A structure that often is pretty similar for many songs in that specific genre of music.

Notes are grouped together in phrases to help give them meaning. Just like a sentence forms a thought in writing, a phrase forms a thought in music.

A phrase will finish with a cadence, which can be strong or weak. It has what feels like a beginning and an end, or a setup and a resolution. It builds up some tension that is later released. If a phrase is like a sentence, a section (verse or chorus i.e.) is like a paragraph. Just like a sentence has some kind of theme for it, a phrase also does. And the section has a more overarching theme, and often comes with a greater feeling of resolution.

Some phrases aren't complete by themselves. They feel unfinished. Just like a sentence can feel unfinished if it leaves us hanging. If I write:

"I really like it when…"

It doesn't feel finished. It begs for a continuation. This is what happens when a musical phrase finishes with a weak cadence. It feels unfinished.

A complete musical thought on the other hand will finish with a strong cadence. It will feel resolved.

*"I really like it when,
I get invited to dance. "*

The first phrase feels unfinished. The second one feels finished. When two phrases are put together and the first finishes with a weak cadence and the second with a strong, it is called a period. Phrases within a period can sometimes feel like a question and answer.

PART THREE - MUSICALITY AND DANCE

Music is Time-Based

All music is time-based. If there is no time, obviously, there is no music. But I would also like to say that if it doesn't change over time, there is no music. When we talked about a definition of music, we learned that it is often contrasted with noise and randomness. If noise is unpleasant, then we can assume that music should be pleasant. And only a constant beat, like a hammer banging with a constant beat doesn't really live up to that criteria in my opinion. Let's see:

1	2	3	4	5	6	7	8
•	•	•	•	•	•	•	•

Very structured and nice looking maybe, especially if we have OCD. But if I want to dance to it, it doesn't look very interesting. Just eight hits with the hammer. Just a constant beat. It is danceable? Yes. If we only want to take eight heavy steps. Is it stimulating? No. Does it give many options to play with musicality? Not so much.

But, if we would use the same hammer, hammering with a rhythm that changes over time, it could be considered music.

What about this:

1	2	3	4	5	6	7	8
•	•	•		•	•	•	

We have some pauses. A little better, right? If you dance salsa, no doubt you recognize this. This change means we can also do some pauses in our moves. Or, if we prefer, we could do something slower in that pause. We could extend the moves we do on 3 and 7 to cover two beats. We would do two normal moves, then a slow move, then two normal and then a slow. One, two, threee, five, six, seveeen. A bit more interesting than the constant beat, if you ask me.

Another example could be if we add something more in there, in between beats. So, we would bang with the hammer twice in one count. Then normal tempo, then twice again and so on.

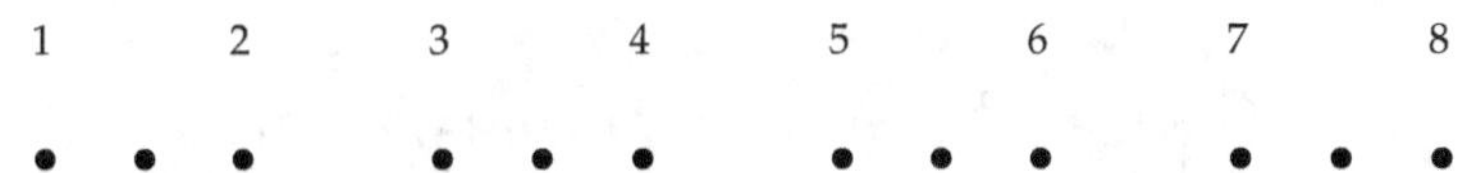

One and two, three and four, five and six, seven and eight. In a way, this is the same as the previous one, only faster. Here we also get something more to play with. We can change our moves to play more with the timing. Two fast steps and then normal. Two fast steps and then normal, and so on.

And if we combine these two tempos in a new way:

Ooone, three and four, fiiive, seven and eight. We are getting even more to play with.

In these examples there is only one "instrument". With a hammer we can't play with the duration of the sound, but we could play with the duration in our dance.

And when we have real music the possibilities to play with the music are almost endless. There are many more instruments and much more variability. But remember, if it doesn't change over time, there is no music. Or, at least not very pleasant music.

Dance Needs to be Time-Based

So, if we want to dance to music, which is time-based and changes over time, we need to change how we dance over time too. We need to change during a song, and of course, since all songs are different, we also need to change how we dance from song to song. If we are always dancing in the same way, no matter the music, we are not really dancing to the music. We are just executing moves with our bodies, and the music is in the background like a kind of soundtrack, but without having any effect on how we dance.

Learning how to execute moves is easy. Learning how to really dance is more difficult. We don't want to dance the same way all the time. We want to mirror the music. We want to create emotions. And sometimes we want to surprise.

The connection between music and dance is essential. So, what is dance, really?

Is it possible to dance without music? Yes, we can move without music and call it dancing. I think so. And we can put music on and move. But if we don't move with the music it doesn't make much sense. We could just as well turn the music off, because we don't use it. The dance might even look better without the music since the moves are not matched to it anyway.

Even if we can dance without music, dance is normally something we do with the music. Music and dance coexist symbiotically. Dance becomes much better with music. And if you are a dancer, music becomes better with dance.

The music is our script. It will tell us what to do, if we just listen. With only steps on the beat we will never follow the music because we are missing out on the bass, the melody, the dominant feeling of the song, and all the other instruments and accents.

Moving without any regard to the music playing doesn't make much sense. Just like music is often contrasted to noise, dancing without any connection to the music playing might look like what noise sounds like. If we see two dancers side by side, one is musical, and one is not very musical, then we will understand why musicality is important. If there is no connection between music and dance it will seem disconnected. It almost becomes disturbing to watch, just like noise can disturb us when we hear it.

Having good technique doesn't mean that we are really dancing. Dancing requires musicality. And it is only when we really listen to the music and express it in our movements that we start dancing.

Our inspiration for moves must come from the music playing, so that our bodies represent something in the music.

The Physical Representation of the Music

When we dance, we are the physical representation of the music that is playing. Our moves should be a reflection of the music. The moves should represent something in the music - they should mirror the music somehow. We have to play with the rhythm, the melody, the accents, the dynamics, and more to create our dance.

Since we are the physical representation of the music, we could imagine someone being able to "hear" the music from the moves that we do, even if they couldn't hear the actual music. Or expressing it another way, someone should be able to "see the music" in our dance. A person watching a long and slow move would see what a longer duration sound in the music sounds like. Let's take an example:

Imagine lifting the right arm out from the body so that it is horizontal, straight out to the side. From there we slowly swing it from the right to the left in front of us. Yeah, let's do it now!

What would that move sound like? Just imagine a sound.

Or, if we take another example:

Imagine if we turn our head quickly from left to right and then back. Repeating the move over and over. What would that move sound like? Just imagine it.

In these cases, we made a move with the body and imagined what that move would sound like.

When we dance, we already have the music. We already have all the sounds. So, we have to reverse it. When we dance, we have to give moves to those sounds instead. A long swoosh. What would that look like?

And a "tic toc tic toc". What would that look like? Yeah, those sounds could have been the inspiration to the two moves we just did, with our right arm and with our head. If we make the swoosh at the same time as we swing our right arm in front of us it makes sense. It sounds right. Or if we make the "tic toc tic toc" at the same time as we turn our head repeatedly from left to right and then back. It also makes sense.

Imagine the opposite. We swing our arm, but do the "tic toc" sound? It doesn't make sense. Or we do the head turns and make the swoosh sound. It also doesn't make sense.

Musicality for dancers is how we hear the music, how we interpret it and then express it in our dance. What sounds are there? Which sounds do we choose to dance to? And how do we express those sounds with our body?

There are many different aspects of this. Most of the skills we will cover are part of that universal language we talked about before. They make sense. When we really listen to the music, we will be able to hear and understand this language. And then it comes down to writing our own story using the words we get from the music. We add our personal interpretation and create our own dance.

PART FOUR - NINE SKILLS IN MUSICALITY

This upcoming part of the book is in a specific order because that is the only way to write a book, in some kind of order. There has to be some order to the sentences, paragraphs, sections, and chapters. This doesn't mean that I believe that the order it is written in is the order that all people have to learn musicality. But I do believe that the first skill is necessary to become really good at most of the other skills.

Most dancers are good at using some of these skills, and not so good in others. So, the same dancer can be very advanced playing with different tempos, but a beginner finding the dominant feeling of a song for example.

I am not claiming that this is the one and only complete list of musicality skills. To me, the list has been growing over time, also since I started writing this book, and I think it will continue growing. So, it is a work in progress. My theory of musicality for dancers. It includes both what I teach on a consistent basis in my live workshops around the world, and quite a lot that I rarely have time to teach.

- *The First Skill* -
Dancing to the Beat

The first skill in musicality is basically to be able to find the beat and move on it, no matter whether it is steps on the ground or moves with other parts of the body. For all dances we normally step or move on the beat. And when we talk about steps, we talk about the weight change. The step doesn't happen when the foot touches the floor. It happens when the weight change occurs. It is like an instant in time, and this instant needs to be exactly on the beat.

When we step a bit too early or a bit too late, we are off time or off beat. If we want to look good when we dance, or look even decent, then we really need to get this right. We need good timing.

If we return to our translation metaphor, being able to dance to the beat is just as essential for a dancer as it is for a translator to have good pronunciation. We can have a great vocabulary and know all the grammar in a foreign language, but if we have truly horrible pronunciation people will still not understand. It is the same with timing. If timing is off, nothing that we do on the dance floor will look really good.

And to get the timing right there are two things we need to do. We need to find where this beat is, and we need to coordinate our moves to it. I really believe that getting this right is fundamental to be able to express anything to the music. And if we are unable to find the beat and get the timing right, we will not be able to do much else either. It has to be automatic, or we will be too focused on it to be able to do anything else.

A Note About Counting

Dancing to the beat doesn't mean that we have to know how to "count" in the music. We don't necessarily need to know where one or five is if we just want to find the beat and dance to it. But if we dance couple dances where there are also rules on which count we step on then we will also need to find out where in the music we are. We need to figure out the 8-count.

Figuring this out can also be good to better understand music in general, to find out where in the music something is happening, as well as for some other musicality skills.

But it is important to remember to not "count" with the whole body. Counting can go on in the head, but we shouldn't show it in our bodies.

And too much focus on counting or finding where the one is might make all our moves seem disconnected. We might look very stiff and there is no flow.

With better and better musicality, the need to count will disappear. We will develop a feeling for the music and it will come naturally. And the flow in our moves will become better.

Moving to the Beat is Natural

Some people claim to have two left feet, meaning that they can't dance. A big part of that is about this skill. They might feel unsure about where the beat is, and/or they think that their timing is not right. But, if we want to dance, there is absolutely no reason not to try.

Nodding our head to the music, humming along or tapping the foot to the beat is probably some of the easiest and most common ways we hear music and express our musicality. Quite often we even do it without thinking.

Finding the beat and moving on it is something that some people can do immediately, and others will have to struggle a bit more to get right. But I believe anyone can do it. It is just about creating some coordination between the mind and the body. And doing that just requires practice.

In some genres of music it is easier to feel the beat, and in others it is more difficult. There can be more happening in the music, like a higher tempo, several rhythms going on at the same time, and there can even be changes in this beat over time. This can all make us confused about what to listen to.

Before we are used to hearing the beat, it will be a bit more difficult to dance, because it might all sound the same. Too many sounds at the same time, which makes it hard to figure out what to move to.

How to Dance to the Beat

Finding the Beat

Hearing the beat is something that we are born to do. Listening to a lot of music, and just trying to stomp the feet, clap the hands, snap the fingers or tapping the hand on the table and we will get it with time. But it is not entirely logical to hear the 8-count. It is quite a bit about feeling.

When it comes to finding the beat, the most reliable part of the music is the percussion. The beat is usually present in the percussion of a song.

But we will sometimes get the first indication of the tempo and where the beat is before the percussion starts, already in the intro of a song. The first ten seconds can tell us. Other times it will take a bit longer. The more we listen to music, the faster and easier it will be to find the beat. And once we find it we can be pretty sure this tempo will continue throughout the song.

Finding the beat will come with time, and when we try to find the one, there are some clues we can use to help:

- Listen for a beat with more emphasis (louder, stronger, etc) than the others. Quite often the one and the five have a bit more emphasis, and the one usually has a bit more than the five. This is not always the case. Sometimes the beats have similar emphasis.

- Within an 8-count the first measure is sometimes called the heavy measure and the second is called the light measure. Some music will transmit this feeling, where the first four counts will have a heavier feeling than the second part.

- Listen for the downbeat and upbeat. This is a two-beat pattern, usually coming from the drums. The downbeat is usually heavier or deeper (boom), while the upbeat feels lighter or higher (ka). As if we did a stomp with the foot and then a clap with the hands or snap with the fingers. Most of dance music has this structure, even if it can be quite in the background. So, in an eight count it would be like 1 (boom), 2 (ka), 3 (boom), 4 (ka) and so on. The emphasis on down- and upbeat varies, and it is not fool proof, but it can help us when we navigate the 8-count.

- Vocals or the melody *can* lead us right, but they can also lead us wrong and confuse us, as they are not always sung on the beat and don't always start on one. So be aware of this. Quite often it matches up nicely, but sometimes it can confuse us a bit. It can also often help to listen to the words in the song, for the finish of a sentence. Or to listen for the natural breathing pauses of the singer. Quite often there is a 1 coming up on the first emphasised beat after that. But don't rely on vocals alone. It is too uncertain.

- Listen to a phrase in the music and try to feel the set-up and resolution. It will often stand out in some way. The first measure (1-4) will feel more like a start, and the second (5-8) will feel more like a finish. After the resolution, you would find a 1 coming.

- Listen for the beginning or end of a section, like the verse or chorus. When these changes take place, instruments often start or stop playing and the first beat of a new section can be even more emphasised. And in the end of a section it can often be even clearer than when a phrase finishes because the resolution will be greater. It can finish with a break, or maybe with extra percussion.

Finding the one is not science. There are no absolutely clear rules. But using these tips, taking them all together and listening to a lot of music we can develop a feeling for it.

Timing

Timing is about how good we are at matching our moves to the music. How well we are able to start and finish our moves on time. If we want to make a move to one specific sound, we need to both start and finish the motion at the right moment to match it well to the music. The transfer of weight needs to come on the beat of the music. This makes it look like we really move to the music. Of course, this applies to all moves, not just steps, even if there is no weight transfer involved, the movement has to start and stop in time to match the music.

If we have never really used our bodies much for movement, if we have spent our life fine-tuning other skills, it might be hard in the beginning. We might have pretty bad timing. But it is just a matter of time - a matter of creating some new connections in the brain. Finding the beat and being able to move to it is the first step to become more musical. Getting this mind-body connection that we need is fundamental to be able to express the music in any way that makes sense. Without it, moves will not come at the right time, they will not come with the right speed or finish on time.

We might start moving too late, when the music is already on its way. Then we will look too slow. And if we start on time but arrive too late, it is also not good. Or if we make a move and arrive too early, it will also look strange. We are not expressing the music in the right way. We would be chopping up the music, stopping before the music stops.

The Beginner Mistake

When beginners dance, they often look stiff and not quite on time. They might look a bit like they are marching, marking the beat a bit too much. A big part of this is because of one fundamental error they do. They move the foot before they move the body.

When we walk, we don't start with the foot. We start the movement by "falling" forward, and then we just let the foot follow. We start with the torso. It is the same in dancing. There might be specific steps or moves that break this rule, but in general we follow this rule in all dances. The foot follows the torso.

If we want to step with our left foot on the beat, we need to start the motion before. So maybe half a beat before we are supposed to finish the move, we would start in the direction we want to go. The right foot presses into the floor and gives us the direction, the left foot follows and we step with it, arriving on time, on the beat.

So, we have to remember this if we struggle with timing. We first start moving our torso in the direction we want to go, and then we follow with the foot. This is true for couple dancing too, in all cases where we should lead more with the frame than with the arms. It makes following much easier when the lead starts with the body before the foot moves.

For other types of moves, the same rule applies. If we want to finish the move on time, we need to start it before.

To get the timing right this is the most important tip there is. And from there it is just one thing we have to do. Dance a lot. It will come gradually, with time, and most of all with practice.

Exercises

Perception

- ‣ Pick three popular songs and listen to the music. Pay attention to the beat and try to find the correct 8-count.

Listen if you can hear the down- and the upbeat. Listen to what distinguishes the 1 from the other beats. Also try to find the difference between 1 and 5.

Expression

▸ Pick a song from your dance genre. Pay attention to the beat and start moving to it, either with your hands, your feet, or your body. Try to really keep the same beat as the music and move so that you start and finish the movements in sync with it. If you are new to this and your own dance genre is difficult, try with some simple electronic dance music which often has a beat that is quite easy to pick up.

- The Second Skill -
Dancing to Different Tempos

The second musicality skill is about changing tempos to the music. It is often something that people usually manage to get pretty fast, at least in simpler moves. But there is also a big problem with it. And we will come to that problem in just a bit.

If we look back at our translation metaphor, this is maybe similar to intonation. When something is translated to a different language using the wrong intonation it can sound a bit off. We understand what is said, but it just doesn't sound right. Dancing to different tempos can be the same. If it is not done right, it can look a bit off.

The most common ways of changing tempo are from the normal beat we usually use when we start dancing to either slow (half tempo) or fast (double tempo). Sometimes, the tempo can be even slower. And especially in solo dances, it can also be even faster.

Timing is still just as fundamental, and it is more difficult to get the timing right when we start playing with different tempos. Now we need to be just as good with timing, but the tempo we do it will vary. It will require more control of our movement. Some moves will be fast, and some will be slow, but we still need to both start and finish just in time. Not too fast and not too slow.

Using Different Tempos

So, if we have eight beats and if we do slow moves (half tempo) during these eight beats we would take four steps or do four moves. Half tempo for eight beats is 8 / 2 = 4 moves. If we would do fast moves (double tempo) on all eight beats we would do 16 steps or moves as 8 * 2 = 16.

I would say it is very rare that we move 16 fast moves in a row. Four slow moves in a row might be more common, but since music changes over time, we would not be dancing this way for very long.

Some parts of a song might fit better with syncopations and other parts might be better with slower moves. The music will change over time. So, we have to adapt to that.

A Problem with Different Tempos

A problem that can come along with this second musicality skill is that some get stuck on it. We start playing around with these different tempos. We think we are done, that we have figured musicality out. Or we get so fascinated by this concept of different tempos that we forget to move past it. We forget to listen to other aspects of the music, and we don't develop the other skills in musicality.

As there is a leader in couple dancing, it is the leader who mostly decides what in the music to dance to and how to express it. And it is also normally the leader who is the one most responsible for getting stuck.

When leaders get stuck playing with tempo changes it is also quite common that they are stuck in either doing un-proportionally many slow moves, or un-proportionally many fast moves. Maybe doing too many fast moves is more common. It seems to be more fascinating. It is as if the capacity to hear anything else disappears. But the problem with too many slow moves also exists.

This problem with getting stuck is part of why many followers complain about leaders not listening enough to the music. The leaders start dancing on the beat, get better, progressing from just dancing on the beat to playing with different tempos in the music. It is a huge improvement, no doubt. They have slightly better technique and musicality than before, but they still hear only part of the music and often exaggerate that part. They can hear more variation, but they are still not really listening. And it often takes a long time to move on. Some never do.

So, they dance the same no matter what feeling a specific song is meant to portray. They still don't listen to the music as a whole, and they don't change their dancing to fit each song. It is like they only have one speed setting in their body.

This can be a bit tricky to explain. Because it can be that they are technically right. There might be something in the music that says, "do a syncopation here". And it will fit well to do a syncopation if we listen to that specific instrument. But, and here comes the tricky part, there can also be something in the music that tells us to do something else. And this is what is often missing - the feeling of when it is right to do it and when it is not. "One speed dancers" have this selective hearing. If we have a tendency like this, that we listen more to some aspects of the music and less to others, then we can try to make an effort to listen more to what we usually don't listen to. We can practice getting more variability in what we listen to and what we express. And we can also look for that feeling when it is right and not. The next skill is where we try to figure out how to really fix it.

How to Dance to Different Tempos

First of all, we have to decide what in the music we want to express. Of course, it only makes sense to do something fast when there is something fast in the music. And the same goes for slow. So, we need to listen to this and once we know we need to prepare for it.

If we have a certain tension in the body when we move to the normal beat, and then want to do something faster, we simply need to create a bit more tension throughout the body. From core out to the legs and arms.

If we have a partner, we also need to make our partner understand this. Thanks to the rule of matching body tension, followers usually learn to respond to the tension. They will give the same tension back as what they receive in the frame. This has to be done just a little bit before, so we prepare our partner for the fast move. If we are solo dancers, we know what will happen and we don't need to prepare our partner. We just need to adjust our own tension.

The actual fast moves are no rocket science. We do the same moves we normally do, but faster. There is one very important difference though. We might need to make the moves a bit smaller. A long step will take more time than a small step. So, if we want to make a fast step, it might have to be smaller. This is true for any kind of move. The size of it has to be adapted to the tempo we want to make it in.

If we want to do something at a slower tempo we don't need to relax more, unless we also want to make something that requires more flexibility. But if we dance a couple dance, we might need to control our partner more, to make sure we stay together. This might sometimes require a bit tighter frame. We need to send the signal that we are going to slow down. So, a tighter frame might work a bit in the same way a seat belt does. It keeps the follower close to us when we slow down. Of course, this doesn't mean that we squeeze our partner. Just making our frame a bit tighter sends enough of a signal to slow down.

And once we are done with the tempo change, whether it is faster or slower, we can go back to a normal body tension.

When we start out playing with different tempos, we can try to focus only on weight changes first and forget about the direction of the step. We can basically just stand in place and make weight transfers, getting the rhythm pattern into the body before we add the direction of the move. This helps to better connect to the music, especially for beginners. The direction has no connection to the music, but the rhythm does. If we want, we can even add our own counting of the tempo as an auditory cue before we start with the rhythm pattern. That way we would have established the rhythm before we start moving.

Exercises

Perception

- ‣ Pick a song from your dance genre and listen to it. Where is it better to move to the beat? Where are there good opportunities to dance on double tempo? Where are there good opportunities to dance on half tempo?

Expression

- Record yourself dancing and then watch the recording. Do you dance mostly on tempo or do you have a tendency to hear the faster or slower tempos more? Whatever tendency you have, try to listen to the music and focus more on the tempo you used *less* in your recording.

- *The Third Skill* -
Finding the Dominant Feeling

The third skill in musicality is about finding the dominant feeling. Other words to describe it could be finding the meaning of the music or the essence of it. If we don't get this right, there will always be something missing in our dance. Something that will look a bit off.

Reproduction of Dance Versus Production of Dance

In my opinion, this skill is missing quite a lot on the dance floor. Partly because of people getting stuck on using different tempos. But probably also because dance (at least couple dancing and the world within couple dancing where I come from) is often taught as reproduction of dance. People are mostly taught fixed patterns. They are taught how to do long sequences, without much regard to the music.

I see several problems with this. One is that they focus on learning long sequences instead of technique. Sometimes in class, the followers know the steps before the leaders do, and just do them on autopilot. And a problem for leaders with learning long sequences is that they will focus on them when they dance. They will try to remember and do them step by step. And then they dance by connecting different long sequences together. At the end of one sequence, they start thinking of what sequence to do next. And then they do that one. Finishing in the same way again, thinking of what to do next over and over again. When this happens, there is never a thought in the moment where a dancer is listening and adapting to the music. They will not learn how to listen to it. There is never any creation of their own dance, because all they do is repeat what someone else has taught them, putting together a mix of other peoples' dance.

When there is no room in the mind for listening to the music there is even less of a chance that they will adapt the dance to it. And good luck on creating something new. It would be better to learn technique, musicality and how to combine it in different ways to create their own dance.

This long sequence dancing is reproduction of dance as opposed to production of dance, where a dancer produces their own dance to the music. It is far too common that dancers reproduce someone else's dance, doing exactly the sequences they have learned in class, instead of creating something of their own. Sometimes it is possible to see which teacher is the big inspiration to someone on the dance floor because they do a lot of the moves that this specific teacher does.

I am not saying it is wrong to take inspiration from someone. I am not saying people shouldn't have their favorite style and try to dance that way. I am just saying that dance is richer when it is our own, when it is not a carbon copy of someone else. When we just copy someone, we lose our creativity. I think it is better to create our own style or our own flavor of dance.

So, I don't believe that musicality is about copying someone else's dance. It is not about doing long sequences of steps that someone taught us.

Real dancing is something more. We need to really listen to the music and chose what moves to do in this moment. We cannot keep stitching together sequence after sequence. We need to be present and, in each moment, find what to dance to. And we need to figure out that thing that really connects our dance with the music. It is not just finding the beat. And it is not just doing faster or slower moves. There is something in each song that tells us how to dance. There is still something missing.

The Dominant Feeling

Yes, there are some things that we can, objectively, do right when we dance. We could step on the beat, we could dance on double tempo when there is something in the music that tells us we can do it, and we could do a slow move when there is something slow in the music.

We could even explain everything, justify why we do them, pointing to something in the music that they were meant to express, but we would still not be getting the musicality right. Why is that?

Some music sounds happy. Some sounds sad. It can be about love or hate, sorrow or happiness. There are many different feelings that music can express. Besides these literal feelings we can also search for how the music sounds. Some music sounds very sharp with a kind of staccato feeling. Some sounds very soft and fluid. Some have high energy, and some have low.

Some of these are things we have to search for and try to feel, and others we can figure out if we understand the lyrics.

If we return for a second to our translation metaphor, the dominant feeling could be something similar to using literal translations versus finding the right expression and getting the tonality right. Some things will come out rude if we translate literally, word for word from one language to another, without getting the tonality right. Some things will be possible to understand, but will still sound very weird, because there is an idiomatic expression that is always used in the target language. People will maybe understand, but it might sound very strange to them.

It is the same with the dominant feeling if we don't get it right – it is possible to dance, but it might feel very strange.

There are many different aspects of this dominant feeling. It covers many different things, and most of them are not either on or off, they are on a scale, like a volume control. It is not happy or sad. We have everything between happy and sad, between sharp and fluid, and between high and low energy. Everything in music is on a scale. Quite literally.

Listening to all these aspects and more, and merging them into something whole is what I call finding the dominant feeling of a song. When we find it, we will know how to dance to that song.

Will we dance more on a slower tempo or a faster tempo? Half tempo (two beats per move) or double tempo (two moves per beat) or something else? Will we dance with a lot of energy, or not so much energy? Will we make big steps and moves or small steps and moves? Will we move the body a lot, or be a bit stiffer using a more restricted movement? Will the body move in a sharper way or a softer and more fluid way?

Changes Over Time

The dominant feeling is something that often stays pretty much the same in a song. There can be different parts that have different feelings, there can be breaks and crescendos, there can be intros and outros that feel different than the verse and the chorus, but the general feeling of a song is often pretty similar throughout a song. It reflects something that the musician wanted to express for that piece as a whole, and for different parts of that song as it changes over time. The most obvious changes can be heard in a break or a crescendo for example, but phrases where a new instrument starts or stops playing can also change the feeling.

When we catch this dominant feeling, we will still need to listen to the changes over time and change how we dance to reflect it well.

The music might not be composed specifically for dancing, but there was some kind of feeling the musician wanted to communicate. Some kind of energy. And we will find it, if we really listen for it.

When we find this feeling and are able to show it in our dance, we have come a very long way. If we can move on the beat with good timing, play with different tempos and also dance to the dominant feeling, very few partners would complain about lack of musicality.

But it can be rare. A lot of people will dance exactly the same to all songs, only changing the speed of their dance to adapt it to the BPM. They do all the same moves that they always do, just at a slightly slower or higher pace. Others might also use changes in tempo. Some might even use other musicality skills. But if we miss this dominant feeling there will be something that both looks and feels off in our dance. The dance is not connected to the music. It will not look like the music sounds.

How to Find the Dominant Feeling?

In my opinion, catching this dominant feeling is one of the most important aspects of musicality. It is a skill that is a bit like "make it or break it". Just like timing is fundamental to make any dance look good. Finding the dominant feeling is fundamental to making dance to a specific song look good. We can't be too far off.

And to catch it we need to choose what moves to do. Some moves fit better with some music. Some music is sharper for example, so it will fit better with sharper moves.

The second thing we need to do is choose how to do it. It will not make sense to dance in a very happy way when the music is sad and mellow, singing about broken hearts. Conversely, it will make sense to make our moves softer if the feeling is soft.

Luckily, we don't have to be great dancers to be able to do these things. So, it is actually possible for a beginner to catch this feeling and really dance to the music, even if he or she doesn't really have that great technique or know that many moves yet.

When we first start learning how to catch this dominant feeling, we might have to consciously think about it. If we are not used to paying attention to it, if we normally just start moving and do what we always do, then we need to focus on it. We need to pay attention. So we can think - what is it that this music tells us?

- What is the melody like?
- Is the music sharp or soft?
- What tempos are more dominant in this music, is it half tempo, on tempo, or double tempo?
- How does it feel, is it happy or sad?
- Is it high energy or low energy?

There are many different aspects to this. These are some questions that can help us find it. But in general, it is about feeling. Finding a way to move that fits the feeling in the music. If we understand the words, it will help us find this feeling.

Is it Sharp or is it Soft?

First of all, we need to be able to make a decision on what kind of moves fit with this music. If it is very soft music it doesn't make sense to make very sharp moves.

If the music is sharp on the other hand, it is better to pick other types of moves which give that sharp feeling. If the music sounds very sharp it will look strange to do a lot of soft moves. This is one way of better catching the dominant feeling.

And just like the sharpness of a song tells us what kind of moves to do, and to skip some moves, it can also tell us *how* to do the moves we still do.

If the song is very soft and fluid, we need to adapt the leading and following to fit that feeling. Let's say we choose a pretty normal move, neither very sharp nor fluid. We can still adapt it more to the music by changing how we do it. If it is a soft and slow song, we make the move softer. We could relax the body more and make all moves more connected. For sharper music we would have to change our bodies and engage our core a bit more. If we want to move quicker and more direct, we need to be prepared. And we are prepared when we are a bit more tense in the body.

We can make these kinds of changes in any move we make. One change could be the way we take our step. Every step we take we also move the body in some direction. There is a transition of weight. How can we increase the sharpness of a step?

In my classes I often make a demo where I play a certain song and I dance to it in two different ways. I ask the students to tell me which way they prefer. I try to move in exactly the same way with my body, but I make one change with my feet. In the first demo I do I move my feet in a normal way. The step comes as it normally does. The weight shift comes as it normally does.

In the second demo I do I try to take my step faster. I keep the feet close to the ground and move the feet fast into position and then my body comes a bit later. The actual step is faster, the foot spends less time moving, and more time on the ground. And the body weight transfer comes when it normally would. This makes the step seem sharper, since it comes faster.

Most students notice this change and usually say they prefer the second demo because it fits better with that specific song I chose. This way of stepping fits well with songs that have a sharp beat because the sharp step looks more in tune with the music.

We can make the same kind of adjustment with pretty much any move we make. If the music is soft and fluid, the body moves in a softer way, more relaxed. If the music is sharper, we need to change in the opposite direction. We need to engage the core a bit more. Our movements might have to be a bit more tense, more direct, and a bit quicker.

Is it Happy or Sad?

Some music sounds very happy, and some sounds sad. Some music doesn't express any strong feeling. If we understand the language, the lyrics will make it a lot easier to pick up on this feeling, but when we don't understand, we just have to guess.

Of course, it doesn't make much sense to dance in a very happy way to music that sounds sad. And it doesn't make much sense to dance in a sad way to happy music.

So, this is something else we have to take into account in our dancing when we try to figure out the dominant feeling of a song. What mood does it give us? How does it make us feel? How can we express that in our dance? How can we change the way we move to reflect that?

Is it High Energy or Low Energy?

Some music is very energetic and can make even the sleepiest person wake up. Other music will almost make us fall asleep. Remember that the energy is not the same as the BPM. It can definitely affect it, and I would say it usually does. But a song with a high BPM can also have a low energy. And a song with low BPM can have a high energy.

The energy level of the music tells us how to dance too. With high energy we might want to express more movement. Maybe we move around more on the dance floor. Maybe we make bigger moves alone or together with our partner. What does the music tell us to do? Does it just inspire small movements, or is it more energetic and inspire big moves?

What Tempos Dominate?

One of the most important parts of catching the dominant feeling is to decide what tempos are good to use to the music we hear. Does the song inspire us to dance more on half tempo and tempo? Is it mostly just on tempo? Or is it more on tempo and double tempo? Or does it have a lot of variability, where we use everything - double tempo, tempo, half-tempo, and maybe even super slow?

And what is it that influences this decision?

Super Slow

Usually when we are inspired to dance really slowly (4 counts or more per move) it is because there is either a break or there are sounds in the background that have a very soft and fluid feeling, and also a long duration. It could be some strings or synthesizer pads. Or it can be the singing, syllables which drag on for four or more beats.

This inspiration to dance more slowly can come even if there is a pretty strong beat and even if there are pretty obvious possibilities to also dance on a faster tempo, with syncopations. But it is common that these longer duration sounds take over and dominate the faster percussion.

Slow - Half Tempo

The slow moves (half tempo) are often because of the vocals, or some heavy bass with longer duration. This heavy base is very common in many songs and therefore we can often use it. It often comes once or twice in a count of eight, and in songs which are not heavily dominated by a specific tempo we can use them to create more variation in our dance and the tempos we dance on.

On Tempo

The normal tempo on the beat is often on some form of percussion, the drums. This tempo is probably what is most common, what most people use in their dance. And it is also what is rarely wrong. It is the safest bet in a way. But it is also one that is not really demonstrating much of musicality. It doesn't provide much variation or surprises at all. So, if we want to be considered a musical dancer, we will need to vary our dance and not only dance on tempo.

Fast - Double Tempo

The double tempo is something that is very common in many songs. We often find it in percussion, the vocals or some accent. Since it is so common it is possible to use this quite a lot. The possibility is there, but it might still not be the best choice if we want to dance to the dominant feeling. Why? Because there is often something else in the music telling us to do something slower. The base, some strings or pads in the background or the vocals can call for moves that are slower. They ask the dancer to do some slower moves, even if there are also instruments playing with double tempo at the same time.

We can do fast moves anytime there is something fast in the music. But it can sometimes look a bit stressed or not quite right.

When we get inspired to dance faster, more on double tempo, quite often it is not the presence of faster rhythms that inspire us. Rather, it can be the lack of these longer duration sounds from the melody, vocals, or something in the background. When we remove the melody or those longer duration sounds there is nothing left in the music that keep us dancing slower, so these songs will tell us to dance more on tempo and faster.

Within a specific genre there is often the same kind of beat, more or less. What usually makes the difference in what tempo we are inspired to choose is this presence or absence of slower sounds.

It is Ok

In class, I often say that if we have a Ferrari and the speed limit is 50 km/h we might feel like pushing it a bit. We might feel like speeding a bit, testing the limits of the car. In dancing it is the same. If we dance with a follower who is really good, and the music tells us to take it very easy, to mostly just slow dance in a closed position, we might still want to do something more. We might still want to open up and do some more advanced moves. It is ok to do it. The "speed limit" of the song might tell us to take it slow, but we can push the limit a bit. For a while at least.

It is only if we always dance this way, without regard to the music, without paying attention to the dominant feeling, that the followers start thinking that we don't have any notion of musicality. So, we can switch it up sometimes, but in general we should try to follow what the music tells us to.

Melody

The melody is maybe the part of the music that gives us most variability when it comes to playing with different tempos. When there are vocals in music, they often carry the melody. And it is one of the parts of a song that most influence the dominant feeling. When we follow the vocals or the melody, we can go from very very slow to very fast.

When we dance to music without melody, we often lose a lot of this variability. And with less variability in the tempo, we lose a lot of possibilities in our dance.

The melody is often what makes us distinguish one song from another. In a way, the melody can help us make every dance more unique if we listen to it.

If we want to improve our musicality, finding the dominant feeling is fundamental, and listening to the vocals and the melody can help a lot when we try to find it.

Exercises

Perception

- Pick a song from your dance genre. Listen for the dominant feeling. What does it tell you to do? How does it want you to dance? Should it be soft and relaxed? Or very sharp? How is the energy of the song? What is it in this music that makes you want to dance a certain way?

Expression

▸ With the same song you listened to trying to figure out the dominant feeling, think of how you can adapt the moves you pick to fit even better with the song. How could you change your moves to fit better with the music?

- The Fourth Skill -
Expressing Specific Sounds

If the dominant feeling was mostly about the music as a whole, the fourth skill in musicality is about expressing the specific sounds that we hear.

Returning to our translation metaphor, this could be about how we say things. If I want to say "I love you" but I scream it out as if I am crazy, maybe the one on the receiving end will not trust what I say in words. It is hard to trust those words when screamed out like that. It would be better spoken with a soft and loving tone. It is the same when we dance to specific sounds. They tell us how to move, so we have to listen to what they say.

This skill is about perceiving, interpreting, and expressing these sounds as well as possible. And here we have some different aspects to consider.

Sonic Attributes

The sonic attributes are first on the agenda in this chapter and they describe all the sounds we can hear around us.

- Pitch – the frequency of tone.
- Timbre – the tone colour.
- Volume – the loudness of a sound.
- Duration – for how long the sound lasts.
- Location – the specific place the sound comes from.

All of these except for the location can very easily be used when we dance. So, we have four sonic attributes which we really can play with. Let's dive a little deeper to learn some more and see what we can use them for.

Pitch

The pitch is the frequency of the sound waves and the quality of sound which makes some sounds seem "higher" or "lower" than other. Different pitches are all on a scale, quite literally.

The pitch is determined by the number of vibrations produced during a given time period. And this vibration rate of a sound is called its frequency, measured in Hertz (Hz). The higher the frequency the higher the pitch.

When only one note is played it might not be that interesting from a musicality perspective, especially if it is a note in the middle of the scale. It doesn't say that much. It doesn't give that much inspiration. However, on either end of the scale, either very high or very low, it can be more interesting.

And when two or more different pitches are played in sequence it really gets interesting. It is the relation between these notes that make them interesting. If we have two notes where the first one has a low pitch and the second one has a higher pitch, they give different feelings. The different pitches can represent different "heights" in the vertical plane. This gives us the possibility to play with them in our musicality.

How to Use the Pitch

I know that it is common to use the dance floor mostly in a horizontal plane. We move over the dance floor in two dimensions. Forward and back and right and left, and everything in between. But we can also use the vertical plane - up and down. And the change in pitch is an excellent opportunity to do this, to introduce vertical motion and make our dance 3 dimensional.

Imagine the classical scale "do re mi fa so la ti do". It goes up in pitch, right? If we dance to it, can we show it in our bodies? Can the body express this upward feeling physically? Yes, of course.

So, let's do that. Feel free to just imagine it, or to actually do it.

If we bend our knees slightly. And we put our weight on our right leg. Now we start stepping with our left, then right, left, right, and so on. If we do it to "do re mi fa so la ti do", and for every word and step, we also move our bodies a bit upwards. We stretch our knees just a little bit more. Does it fit that scale? Yes. Does it feel a bit ridiculous? Maybe that too! Especially if we do it with an audience.

These eight notes represent a starting point and then seven moves upwards. If we want to represent it with our bodies, each move upwards cannot be that big. We cannot move that much upwards. And guys have to remember that girls who have high heels are already a bit above the ground so they cannot move as much upwards. We have to take that into consideration when we dance. But it is ok if it is small, as long as we create that feeling of upward motion.

I think this is pretty easy to understand. It is pretty intuitive. But just to make it even clearer. Let's imagine once again we have this scale of "do re mi fa so la ti do". Now let's imagine we sing it in the head while running up some stairs. One step up for each note. A starting point and seven steps up. It makes pretty good sense, right?

Imagine instead that we were running downstairs to the same scale. "Do re mi fa so la ti do". Does that make sense? Does it fit the scale we are singing? No, it doesn't. It doesn't make sense. It feels weird to just imagine running downwards to this upwards scale.

But what if we sang the scale backwards and ran downwards? Then it would make much more sense again. I don't know if I can reproduce that scale backward on a whim, but since I have some time, I can figure it out: "Do ti la so fa mi re do". Yeah, it works to do it that way!

Now we know what makes sense to do when we have a change in pitch. But when can we use it? If we want to create a strong upwards feeling when we are playing with the pitch we need to stay in place. When we are moving, taking steps, it is much more difficult to create this feeling. The less we move horizontally, the easier it is to create the feeling of vertical movement. This is something worth remembering when we are playing with the pitch.

This is what pitch is and some examples of how we can play with it, and the changes in it over time. Playing with the pitch is often overlooked. So, we can definitely improve our musicality by adding it to our repertoire.

Timbre

The timbre is the tone color or tone quality and it is what lets us distinguish between different instruments, even if they are playing the same note and volume.

The timbre makes it possible to distinguish between a choir and a piano, between different categories of instruments, such as string instruments and wind instruments, and also between different instruments within each category, such as trumpet and trombone.

The different vibrations of sound waves are pretty complex. Most sounds vibrate at several frequencies at the same time. The extra frequencies are called overtones or harmonics. The relative strength of these helps determine a sound's timbre. Some sounds are very similar in timbre and will be more difficult to distinguish, and some are very different. Besides this, the way we play an instrument can affect its timbre and therefore the sound.

All instruments give sounds that have a certain feeling to them. Some give a very soft and airy feeling. Others are very sharp. Some are very heavy, felt very deeply in the body, like a deep base tone, and others are just barely possible to hear. All these different timbres will affect what kind of moves that make sense to do to them.

Some instruments also vary a lot in how the sounds feel depending on the pitch that is played. They might feel very soft and airy on the higher notes and be much heavier and felt more in the body on the lower notes.

How to Use the Timbre

How can we use the timbre in our musicality? Well, maybe it is not as easy as with the pitch, where we can represent it easily just by moving in the vertical plane. The timbre is a bit trickier, a bit more about feeling.

But just like we talked about previously, since we are the physical representation of the music, we will still need to show the sounds with our bodies.

A sound that sounds soft and airy, we would have to use a soft and airy move, right? It doesn't make sense to make the body tremble to a sound that is soft and airy. But what if it was a deep base that almost made the air around us vibrate? A base so deep that we feel it in our bodies?

Then I think it would definitely both feel right and look right for people watching.

Or if we imagine a harp playing. It often gives a pretty airy feeling. So, we would have to catch that airy feeling in our dance. Or imagine some timpani drums playing. They can often give a pretty dramatic feeling, and also sound very powerful. We would have to catch that feeling. Or a piccolo flute. They are very small flutes, and they also give pretty small sounds in a way. So, it would often make sense to make small moves to the sounds of a piccolo flute.

There are thousands of different instruments. They all have their own specific feeling in the sounds they produce. They can also often have different feelings depending on which pitch is played. And they can even have different feelings to the sounds depending on how that specific note is played. The possibilities are endless.

Pitch was easy. Timbre is more difficult. It is quite a lot about feeling. But it can help to think about how a sound feels. What would it look like if we could "see" it? How could we make someone "hear" this sound from the move that we do, without the music playing?

Volume

The volume or loudness is the third attribute that defines a sound. And it is probably the term that we use the most in daily language. The volume is how loud we perceive a sound and it is measured in decibels. We could say that the volume tells us if the music is "whispering" or if it is "shouting".

How to Use the Volume

What can we do with the volume? Well, just like we are sometimes whispering and sometimes shouting, we could think in the same way about a specific instrument. If it is played with very low volume, like a whisper, it is not very emphasized. So, maybe we should make a smaller move if we do anything at all. If a sound is very loud on the other hand, we might give it a bigger move. The music is "shouting" it, so we might as well emphasize it in our dance too.

We can always use the volume and play with it in our musicality. But just like with the pitch, I would say that if it is isn't very high or low, or doesn't change that much, it isn't that interesting. It doesn't really stand out. It doesn't give that much inspiration.

It is when the volume changes between different notes that it becomes more interesting. It is the relation between the volume of those notes that make them interesting. If we have two sounds where the first one has a low volume and the second one has a high volume it tells us we can do something with that change, we can express it in our dance, to show what is happening in the music.

Volume also has another important role to fill, and we will come back to it later.

Duration

The meaning of the duration of a sound is pretty obvious. It tells us how long the sound lasts. Some sounds are naturally shorter in duration. A kick drum, for example, has a very short duration, and a drummer can't really extend the duration. With other instruments, like flutes, the musician can easily give a longer duration to a note.

How to Use the Duration

First of all, if we decide to dance to a specific sound, the duration of it tells us for how long we can use it. Is it for one beat? Is it just half a beat? Or is it more, two or four? Of course, a sound can have any duration and it can finish at any point in time. It doesn't have to start nor finish exactly on the beat either. But in general, the duration tells us for how long we can use a sound.

The duration also tells us something about the size of that move, especially for the sounds with a short duration. For a sound that lasts for just half a beat or even one fourth of a beat, we don't have time to do a big move. If we dance to sounds with very short duration, we cannot make moves that take a long time to finish. We wouldn't have time. We would constantly finish the moves late and be out of sync with the music.

It would make more sense to do small moves. Then we can finish the move on time and be ready to start the next move to the next sound we choose to dance to.

Sounds with a long duration give us the opportunity to do moves that are both big and small. But if we do a small move to a long duration sound it can be harder to even notice the move, because it is so small and slow. When the duration is long, it might make more sense to make a slower move, but maybe we can increase the size of it a bit so that it becomes more noticeable and "covers" more of the duration of that sound. Another reason to make it a bit bigger is if we have danced on tempo or faster just before. Then we can make the move bigger, so we have the possibility to slow down the momentum. We often need some time and space to slow down.

The duration of a sound can also tell us something about *how* we can make a move. A quick sound with a short duration often needs to be a bit sharper, besides being pretty small.

Playing with different tempos requires adapting the tension in the body, and when we play with different durations for specific sounds it is one aspect of playing with different tempos. When we play with musicality we constantly need to adapt with our bodies if we want to express the music right.

Location

The location of a sound tells us where it is coming from. In real life when we hear a sound, we can usually determine where it comes from - the location. In the real world, sounds can come from all directions, in three dimensions. With someone talking it is obvious. It comes from the mouth. With non-amplified live music, it is also pretty obvious, it comes directly from the specific instrument. But when we listen to pre-recorded music, which is often the case when we are dancing, we are normally limited to left and right speaker. And a lot of music is recorded in a way that doesn't really distinguish between them. Most instruments come equally from left and right. This makes it more difficult to play with the location of sounds on the dance floor.

If we would know the location, we could play with it too. But very often it comes from both speakers. Unless we have a very controlled situation where we know from where a sound comes, we will not be able to use location. So, from now on we will leave this sonic attribute.

How a Sound is Played and Expressed

When we talk about specific sounds and musicality, it is also about catching the way an instrument is played. We have covered some of this previously when we talked about duration and volume. But there is more to this. The way an instrument is played can be related to both the dynamics, or volume, and also to articulation - how long the notes are played and how they are joined together.

Dynamics

Dynamics in music normally refers to different variations of intensity or volume and is usually measured in decibels. We already talked about the volume quite a bit.

But in music notation dynamics are not absolute values, they are relative ones. Other aspects of the sound can also influence the perception of intensity.

Normally the dynamics are described in Italian words like piano (soft), forte (loud), mezzo piano (medium soft), and mezzo forte (medium hard). Then we also have the pianissimo and fortissimo for very soft and very hard respectively, and more exaggerated intensities. There are also words that describe an increasing or decreasing intensity - sforzato or sforzando for increasing and fortepiano for decreasing.

How to Use the Dynamics

Of course, when we dance, all these intensities will influence our dancing. A loud and accented sound might inspire a bigger or more intense move. A very subtle sound, something that is played pianissimo, may inspire us to do a very small and subtle move. Just the same way as increasing or decreasing intensity can call for increasing or decreasing intensity in the movements when we dance.

Paying attention to dynamics will help us express the individual sounds much better.

Articulation

Articulation is about how a musician sounds the notes, and staccato is probably the most well-known of these. Staccato is the shortening of the duration of a sound compared to the written note value. Legato is another type of articulation and it tells the musician to play the notes in a smooth and joined sequence, without separation. So, if something is played staccato it will make it sound harder, sharper and more disconnected, and legato will make it sound softer and more fluid and connected.

Different articulations, from long to short, from connected to disconnected, are:

- *legato* (smooth, connected)
- *tenuto* (pressed or played to full notated duration)
- *marcato* (accented and detached);
- *staccato* (separated, detached)
- *martelé* (heavily accented or hammered)

For a dancer, it makes a lot of sense to listen to and express different articulations. We are not tied to the musical score in the same way as a musician is, but we need to follow the music. The music is our conductor. It tells us how to move. When we really listen to it, we can choose to move the body in a way that is more staccato or more legato to better reflect how the music is played.

How to Use the Articulation

When the music is played legato, we can join our moves more together, more fluid and connected. We can move in a softer way and we can try to create more seamless transitions between steps or moves. We try to fill out the music more. And with staccato, and even more so with martelé, we can choose moves that are sharper, and try to do all moves in a sharper way. We can move more robot-like. More disconnected, just like the music is.

Vibrato

Vibrato is another way of playing a note. The word comes from the Italian word "vibrare" which means to vibrate and this way of playing creates a regular and kind of vibrating sound. It is really just a slight change in the pitch up and down around the note value played.

Vibrato consists of two factors, how much the pitch is changing, and how fast it is changing.

How to Use the Vibrato

When we dance, one obvious way to express a vibrato is to use a body part to "tremble", preferably with the same "vibration" as the vibrato. How closely we can match the vibrato with our bodies depends on our own dance skills. The faster the vibration, the more difficult and the smaller the moves we can allow ourselves to make. The more the pitch changes up and down, and the slower the change in pitch, the bigger moves we can do.

When we learn how to pay attention to and express the sonic attributes and how the notes are played, our dance will become much richer. Adding all these together, we can talk about textures.

The Texture of a Sound

The texture is "the feel, appearance or consistency of a surface or a substance". Air is light. Syrup is gluey. Fur is soft. A concrete wall might feel rough. But we can also use the term texture to describe the sounds in music, and the moves in our dance. All the sonic attributes together with dynamics and articulation give us a "texture". And when we use textures in our dance, we will express the music much more vividly. If we talk about a dancer who dances in a "soft" way, no matter which dance genre, we can all imagine what it's like. That is using a texture to describe how someone dances. But usually when we talk about textures in dancing, it is about describing how to do a single move.

Every step we take and every move we make when we dance, we make it to a specific sound. One single move can be done in many different ways when we use different textures. A different texture gives the move a different feeling. And this move will fit with a slightly different sound. This way we can adapt one move to many different sounds. When we have many different textures we can use for the same move we all of a sudden make it possible to express the music in multiple new ways.

Imagine we have two moves that we put together. It would mean we have just one combination. Now imagine we have five different textures we can apply to those moves. All of a sudden, we have 5 * 5 = 25 different combinations instead of one. The more moves and the more textures we add, this number increases exponentially. Just adding one more texture, and we get 6 * 6 = 36 different combinations. That's eleven more than with just five textures. Or if we add one more move, we get 5 * 5 * 5 = 125 different combinations. Imagine the possibilities to be creative when we play around with different textures! Imagine how much richer the dance, and how much closer it can match the music!

Dance is the physical representation of the music. When we use textures in our dancing, we become better at describing with our bodies what is happening in the music. We make it easier to "see" the music. We paint a clearer picture. A quick and sharp sound needs a quick and sharp move while a long and soft sound needs a long and soft move.

How to Use the Texture

When we use textures, the first thing we need to do is to pick the sound we want to highlight. Exactly what can go into that decision will be covered later on. But, let's imagine we have chosen a sound, now we need to figure out the characteristics of that sound. Here we will take into account everything we talked about earlier, like the pitch, timbre, volume, duration, articulation and so on. Putting it all together we get an idea of how to express this sound. We try to match the texture of the move as closely as possible to the texture of the sound. Should it be soft, sharp, rough?

If we take an example, imagine we have a specific sound. Now how could we describe that sound? Is the pitch high or low? How is the timbre? How long is the duration? How high is the volume? How is this sound played? Is it staccato? Is it legato? These questions give us the clues to find the texture of that sound. And the texture tells us how we make that move.

This type of choice is something we could do for every move we make. Of course, when we dance, we never go through this process like this. It is much more just the feeling. Our experience tells us what to do and we do it on the fly. There is no way we can pick a sound, ask ourselves five or ten questions, and then ask ourselves how the answers to those questions can be connected to how we express the sound in the body. We need to do it much faster than that, but we can practice on textures thinking of some of these things. The first step is to open up the mind to textures. The more advanced we become, and the more music we know, the more we will get the feeling, and the less we will need to think about it. The more it will come naturally.

Exercises

Perception

- Listen to music from your dance genre and pay attention to the melody (if it doesn't have melody, pick another song, even from another genre if you have to). In the melody, listen to the pitch and just imagine following it, moving up and down in the vertical plane to match the pitch.

Expression

‣ Listen to music from your dance genre. In the melody, listen to the durations. Try to dance to them, so you change the tempo of your moves when there is a longer duration and shorten them when there is a shorter duration.

- The Fifth Skill -
Dancing to the Silence

We often think of music as just the sounds, what we can hear. We think of rhythm, melody and harmony. But we have to remember that music is just as much the silence in-between sounds, and how sounds and silence interact with each other.

Taking a look at our translation metaphor, this could be about also using pauses when we talk. A continuous stream of words, without any pauses, can be hard to understand. Normally when we talk, we use small pauses for breathing, showing emphasis, and more. Sometimes we use an artistic pause for greater effect. A translation would have to use the same kind of pauses for the same effect. And of course, there are pauses in music too, so we have to interpret them too.

So, when we dance, we have to use the sounds, but we also have to use the silence. Everything that happens or doesn't happen is part of it. If we ignore the silence our dance might look stiff and boring.

Like mentioned early on in this book, I don't think knowing how to count the music is necessary to find the beat or for musicality in general. It might even make listening to music a bit too rational if we count when what we really need to do is to feel it. But counting can help us understand and better express some aspects of music.

Sometimes counting is needed to really find the right precision in dance. There might be sounds that we want to express which don't happen on any exact beat. Maybe they happen not on seven and not on eight, but somewhere in between. To find the right precision, we might need to count. And then we may find out that it happens just after seven, but not on seven and a half. It would maybe be hard to get it right if we didn't know exactly where it happens.

And sometimes when there are longer breaks, longer silences, the first times we hear the song we might have to count the beats to know when it starts again. So, counting can sometimes be necessary to know what we can do with the music.

Especially when we start using the silence in our dance, we will sometimes need to know.

How to Dance to the Silence

What does silence "look" like? The most obvious answer would be stillness - no moves. Once the break comes and there is some silence, we stop moving. Only when the sound we dance to comes back, we start again. The silence is used as a contrast to the sounds. The stillness is used as a contrast to the movements.

But I think we can also interpret silence in other ways.

It can be just silence, which could be translated into stillness. No movements. But it could also be interpreted as a preparation, or maybe a build-up. If we imagine a break comes at five and the music starts again on the coming one, there are four beats of silence. These four beats are also kind of a countdown to when it starts again. How can we represent a countdown in our dance? How can we represent preparation?

Maybe silence can also be interpreted with a very slow move? A move that is very restricted or held back. Not totally still, but almost. Like a slow extension of the last sound we danced on. Maybe it doesn't have to be very small, but I think it would probably make sense to make it soft and gradual at least.

Something that can help in how to interpret silence in music is thinking of what happened just before, or if we know, what will happen after the silence. Then we can use what we know and play with the contrast. Did the music gradually just fade out into silence? Or was it a very abrupt ending before the silence? I think this could affect which option we choose, if we make a total stop, or if we still make some movement. When does it make more sense to do a total stop - when the music fades out, or when it stops abruptly?

Silence Gives a Lot of Freedom

There can be total silence. And there can also be partial silence, like when the sound or instrument we dance to stops playing. Since there is an absence of sounds when there is total silence, there are no sounds or sonic attributes to relate to. No dynamics or articulation. So, in a way, the total silence gives the dancer a lot of freedom in how to express it. We can make our own interpretation, with our own personal flavor.

We can even add something, as if the body was an additional instrument playing, interacting with the music in a kind of call and response.

Remember, silence is just as much part of the music as the instruments playing. And therefore, we have to pay attention also to the silence in our dance.

Exercises

Perception

‣ Play some music from your dance genre. Are there any breaks where there is total silence? How could you use that silence in the best way? How could you express it?

Expression

‣ Pick one of the songs from above with a silent break, or almost silent break and plan exactly what you want to do with it. Decide how you will express the silence and decide how you transition to and from silence, and then dance it. Then for the same song, pick another way of expressing it and dance that way.

- The Sixth Skill -
Prediction & Preparation

All music is built on repetition & variation. A lot of the things happening in a song will repeat again. And sometimes they will repeat, but with some slight variation.

All music also has some kind of structure. This is great news because it makes music a bit more predictable.

Returning to our translation metaphor, if a good translator knows the topic, he or she can predict a bit ahead of time what will be said and prepare it in the brain. It is possible to be a step ahead and think of how to express something the best way. It is the same in music. If we are aware it can often be predicted. And therefore, we can also prepare for what to do with it.

There is a structure, but unfortunately it can differ a bit, from genre to genre and from song to song. There are no strict rules. We can get surprised sometimes. But even if there are not strict rules, we will still have a lot of help from this structure. Our brains have evolved to recognize patterns. So, we will get better at predicting whether we want it or not.

The Structure of a Song

The song structure is the arrangement of a song, and it consists of different phrases, periods and sections. We have all heard of intro, verse, chorus, solo, outro, and so on. These are all different sections of music.

One of the more popular structures we hear in modern music is often something similar to this:

- intro
- verse
- pre-chorus
- chorus (refrain)
- bridge (middle eight)
- verse
- chorus (refrain)
- outro

There are many other structures, with different repetitions of verse and chorus. There can also be a solo or other section in the song. Nonetheless, most modern and popular music relies on a structure with a verse and a chorus.

Exactly how long one of these sections is can vary. Sections of 16 or 48 beats are pretty common. But a lot of the music we dance to is mostly built on sections of 32 beats and usually stays the same for each section within a song. If we can figure it out early on, we know what we can expect.

Both verse and chorus are usually repeated, while the intro and outro are only played once. The intro often sets the feeling of the song and normally has no lyrics. But there are no strict rules. There can be several instruments playing, and the intro can also consist of only voice, only drums/percussion or something that is played by just one instrument.

The verse is telling the story or the events in a song. It creates the images and the feelings and it often has rhyming lyrics. It almost always appears more than once, and the subsequent times it appears it has different lyrics. The verse builds up the story for the theme of the song.

Not all music has a pre-chorus, but when it has, it is placed after the verse, just before the chorus. It works to connect the verse to the chorus.

The chorus or refrain is what contains the main idea or main theme of the song, both regarding what is expressed in the music and in the lyrics. What is the message? The chorus rarely varies, so this is something that almost always repeats in exactly the same way. And it always has greater musical and emotional intensity than the verse.

Just like the pre-chorus, the post-chorus is not always there. As the name implies it is placed after the chorus and can often have a similar character to the chorus but is slightly different.

The bridge may be just a transition but more often it is a section that contrasts with the verse. It is used to break up the repetitiveness in a song, create some more variation, and keep the attention. It can be in the form of a middle eight, a section with significantly different melody and lyrics. The bridge usually appears in the second part of the song.

The outro is a way of signaling that the song is about to finish. It makes the ending less abrupt than just finishing on the last measure (or bar) of the chorus section for example. There is rarely anything new introduced in the outro. Rather, something from the song may be used as part of it, and the energy generally goes down.

During a song the energy levels are often low during the intro and outro and highest during the chorus.

In summary, the structure will differ a bit from genre to genre and from song to song, but there is always some kind of general structure. And since all music is built on repetition and variation, understanding and feeling this structure will help us in our musicality.

How to Use Prediction & Preparation

Knowing Many Songs

If we listen to a lot of music we will, of course, know a lot of songs. We will know all the songs we listen to. We will know the dominant feeling as soon as a song starts playing. We have already experienced what feelings it gives us. We will know the melody's ups and downs, the longer durations, when there is a break, or where there is an accent. We will know the crescendos or surprising moments in the song. All the songs we know will become easier to dance to. It will be easy to know what kind of moves to do, and how to do them. And since we know what will happen, we can prepare for the specific moves we want to use to highlight the music.

Understanding the Structure

If we listen to even more music, we will start understanding the structure of the music, what is normal for that genre. We will feel what is going to happen in a song, even if we have never heard it before, because we know the structure subconsciously. We can sense when a phrase or section is finishing or about to begin, we can sense when a break will come, and we sense when the accent is about to come again, even if the song is new for us.

Most popular music is structured in similar ways, and the changes are signaled in the music. It can be in the lyrics, something extra or different in the percussion, or some chord changes in the music that send us the signal.

Active Listening

If we listen at the beginning of a song, we will also be able to guess what will happen later, just from paying attention to the first minute of it. Even if it is some genre which we are not familiar with, and we have never heard it before. Within this time frame there is often something, like a first accent, a first break or something similar happening. Because of the repetition we can be pretty sure it will come again. And there will usually be something in the music that sends us the signal. Then we will know and be ready.

Since both verse and chorus are very similarly built, and if we pay attention to this, we will be able to predict the music when they appear a second time. Popular music usually has the same musical notation for each verse. The chorus also uses the same notation. But the difference is that while the musical notation stays the same there are normally new lyrics for the second verse, even if it is sung with the same rhythm. In the chorus, the music and lyrics will usually both stay the same.

Additionally, within a verse for example, the second period will very often be very similar to the first one, in terms of rhythm. So, if we pay attention in the beginning of a song we have never heard before we will often be able to predict what will happen. Both in the already in the second period of the verse as well as in the second part of the song, when the verse and chorus repeats.

Preparation

Thanks to the structure and the repetition we will be able to feel what will happen, not only in all the songs we know, but also most songs from that genre. And paying a little attention in the beginning of songs, we will also be able to find something we can predict will come again.

This is when we really can start playing with the music. Since we can predict what is going to happen, we can also prepare what to do with it, even for songs we never heard before.

And over time we will do it all subconsciously. We don't need to count or actively think about it. We can just feel it. When we do this, we will have some time to think of what to do. And we will also have some time to get into the right position to do it.

It was mentioned earlier, to listen to a lot of music. This is when it becomes really helpful. Once we start listening to a lot of music, we will start understanding the natural essence of all music. We will start feeling the structure of the music and become much better at predicting.

But we also need to spend a lot of time dancing. It is not enough to be able to perceive the music and predict what will happen. We also need to practice our creative skills, what to do with the music we hear, and prepare for it.

Exercises

Perception

▸ Listen to some music from your dance genre and pay attention to the structure. How is each song structured? What parts are there? When do different parts start? For how many counts of 8 and beats is each part? Try to write the structure down.

Expression

▸ Listen to some of your favourite songs from your dance genre. Some song you really know. Then think exactly what you will do with the music at two or more places in each song, maybe a break and an accent, or something that is easy to distinguish and stands out. Then you play that song again and make sure that you are in the right position to do your planned moves. If you have to do something slow, or a syncopation, just before to get into position, you do that. But preferably do it to the music. Just try to be in the right position to do your move when the time comes. And avoid arriving too fast into position so that you have to stand there and wait.

- *The Seventh Skill* -
 Dancing to the Vocals

Dancing to the vocals is really not that different from dancing to any other "instrument". All the same ideas apply in a way. But the vocals are also a bit special. They can carry meaning and are often what makes a song recognizable. They are very varied and rich and are so important for dance that I think they are a special skill in themselves.

Usually the vocals carry the melody in a song. And some people say that dancing to the melody is really what separates an average dancer from an advanced dancer.

The vocals and the lyrics also have many different aspects we can use as a source of inspiration.

They can carry the rhythm. They are extremely variable and has many different durations. They use many different pitches, and each singer has a personal sound - a specific timbre in their voice. We can recognize a singer, and their voice can create a specific feeling. The vocals can have different articulations and even add a vibrato on top. A singer can whisper the words or scream them out. And last but not least, the words carry meaning. They convey emotions. They can even give instructions.

How to Dance to the Vocals

Syllables

The rhythm that the voice gives comes from the syllables, together with the duration of each syllable. A syllable is a unit of pronunciation that has one pronounced vowel sound. Sometimes it is just a vowel, and sometimes it is a vowel with one or more consonants. But vowels that are not pronounced cannot form their own syllable. A syllable can be a complete word, or it can be a part of a word.

If we take an example. Let's imagine part of the lyrics in a song would be something like this:

"I get it."

There are three words, and there are also three syllables. One syllable per word in this case. I-get-it. But if the words would be:

"I understand it."

There are still three words, but there are five syllables. I-un-der-stand-it. In this example, we would probably make five moves if we dance on the vocals.

But a syllable in itself doesn't say give us the full picture. It doesn't tell us how it is sung. So, we don't yet know how to dance. We can decide we will make one move every syllable, but we don't know what rhythm we will have in our dance yet.

And the syllables don't say anything about the pitch they are sung in. If we want to dance on the vocals, first we need to figure out the rhythm.

Durations

The next step is to also add the durations. Once we know the durations, we have a complete idea of the rhythm we need to dance to. Let's say we have lyrics with the words: I like to dance slowly.

Counting the syllables, it would be: I-like-to-dance-slow-ly. As you can see in this example, not all vowels in a word form a syllable. Only the pronounced vowels can create a syllable. And therefore, not all vowels influence the rhythm. In this case both "like" and "dance" have two vowels, but only one syllable since the "e"s are not pronounced in those words.

Anyway, let's say the duration for each of the four first syllables in our example is one beat, and for the fifth syllable, "slow", the duration is three beats. We give the last syllable a duration of just one beat so that we have a total duration of eight. Yeah, I admit, my profession as a dance teacher has influenced me. I have to finish on eight. Even in the gym, if I want to do 12 reps, I count to eight and then I start over and count to four!

Anyway, back to the topic, in this case, it would be like this:

1	2	3	4	5	6	7	8
I	like	to	dance	slo	ooo	oow	ly

Dancing to this, we would do four moves on the beat, and then one move very slowly, with a duration of three beats. And last, we would finish off with one move with just one beat. This is how the syllables, plus the duration can give us the rhythm to dance to when we want to dance to the vocals.

Pitch

When we learned about the different aspects of sound, we talked about pitch quite a bit. If we also listen to the vocal pitch and express it in our dancing, we are really reaching a higher (pun intended) level of musicality. Since pitch is on a scale, we could visualize this with our bodies or some part of our bodies moving upwards with a rising pitch, and downwards with a pitch that goes down, just like we did when we talked about the pitch in general.

Using the pitch in the vocals adds another dimension to the dancing. But, if we were to use the pitch in the vocals all the time in this way, it would be very hard to combine with other moves. Since the melody is constantly going up and down in pitch, it would probably feel a bit exaggerated to do this all the time, and it would be quite difficult to combine with other musicality skills. Just like we mentioned before, playing with the pitch is easier when we are in place. When we don't move around much on the dancefloor in the horizontal plane it is easier mimic the pitch and to create this feeling of vertical motion.

Articulation

Previously we talked about articulation - how a musician sounds the notes. In speech and singing, we talk about it too, but then we mean the formation of clear and distinct sounds in speech. To speak in an articulate way could maybe be similar to playing an instrument staccato. If someone sings in a very articulate way, it would probably make sense to dance in a very articulate way too, a bit more staccato. It would make sense to do more defined moves, maybe be a bit sharper and direct.

On the other hand, if someone doesn't pronounce each word as clearly, if they sing in a fuzzier way, maybe we could call it legato. And we could also match our dance to that feeling. We could dance to the vocals with a bit less tension, a bit more relaxed and with less defined moves. Because it would better match the articulation in the voice.

When we dance to the vocals it makes just as much sense to listen to the articulation as it does when we dance to instruments playing. A singer can play just as much with this as a violinist or pianist can, so a dancer should probably do the same in the dance.

Words of Meaning

Whenever there are lyrics in a song, there are also words to play with. We don't always know what the words mean, because we might not speak the language, but when we do know it, we can also express them on the dance floor.

Previously we talked about the dominant feeling. If we understand the lyrics it helps us catch the dominant feeling, the feeling for the song as a whole, or for parts of the song. But we can also use the words in a different way. Besides using the story of a song to find the dominant feeling we can use short words or sentences and play with them.

Every word has a meaning. We cannot express all words in moves as some kind of charades, but some of them we can.

Sometimes there are words describing shapes or directions. It can be forward or back. For "circles" we can make a circular move. Or when someone sings "up and down" we can move up and down, if we are going to be very obvious here. But we can use pretty much any word or sentence that is possible to show in our dancing.

It can be someone singing "I love you. How could we express that in dance? Maybe we don't even need to do anything special. Maybe we can stop and listen to the lyrics and our partner will understand. Or we can look at them and try to express it in our eyes.

Doing this the right way we can add an extra connection to the music, with the words, at the same time as we might add in some humor in our dance.

Actions

When I talk about actions in the music it doesn't necessarily have to be something done with the voice, but I have included it here because sometimes they are. There are different actions in the music that we can recognize the sounds of. It can be breathing, maybe it is a knocking on a door, footsteps, maybe a laughter or a "yeah" that we can add to our dance, either singing along or miming somehow.

If we bring the music to life by illustrating these same actions that we have in the music we become something more. We become an actor at the same time. We are both a dancer and an actor. We paint an even clearer picture of the music. And once again, if we master this skill we can often add in a lot of humor in our dance.

Exercises

Perception

- Listen to some music from your dance genre. If you don't understand the lyrics, pick a song in a language you understand, and/or search for the lyrics online. Are there any specific words you could express in your dance? How would you express them?

Expression

- Listen to some music from your dance genre and pay attention to the vocals (if there are no vocals, pick another song, or any song with vocals). Try to use the syllables and duration of vocals and dance only to that rhythm.

- *The Eight Skill* -
Breathing with Musicality

Breathing in General

What about breathing? It is one of the first things we do when we are born, and we keep breathing for the rest of our lives. It is fundamental in our lives and therefore it is also fundamental in dance.

If we take a look on our metaphor again, breathing is fundamental if we want to translate something. Without air we cannot even produce sounds. And not breathing at the right times will give a translation a strange rhythm. Without breathing we cannot dance either. We cannot work optimally on the dance floor.

Breathing correctly can improve our technique, our posture, our timing, our balance, and our flow. And on the flip side, forgetting to breathe, as sometimes happens when we are deeply focused in class, on stage, or maybe when we are dancing with that special someone, can limit all of the above. We simply get nervous, tense up, and forget to breathe. And when we forget to breathe, we don't get enough oxygen. And when we don't get enough oxygen, we can tend to become a bit stupid.

The best dancers breathe consciously and add it to their dance technique practice until it becomes second nature. It can improve dancing greatly when done right.

When we breathe through our mouth it is associated with the "fight or flight" reflex. When we breathe through our mouth, we breathe shallow, and air only reaches the upper lobes of the lungs. This can work for anaerobic sprints, like if a dangerous beast was chasing us. But it is not as good for dancing, when we spend many minutes at a time on the floor. It can be good to practice breathing when we are not dancing, to make it second nature. It can also be good to spend a little more time on exhaling the air, to get it all out of the lungs.

If we want to use breathing for our musicality, first of all, we need to make sure we breathe right. We don't all breathe the same way.

When we breathe through our nose our breathing is deeper, usually slower and we get more oxygen. Breathing deeply also helps our mind focus and makes it easier to stay calm. So, we should try to breathe through our nose as often as possible, and only revert to mouth breathing when necessary.

How to Breathe with Musicality

Is it possible to use breathing in dance to express our musicality? I definitely think so. I use it a lot.

When we synchronize our breathing with our partner, we can create incredible experiences of connection, both with the partner and with the music. Specific techniques of breathing (outside of dancing) can even achieve altered states of consciousness.

So, using breathing in our dance can definitely enhance our dancing. But what can we do to connect the breathing to the music and express our musicality?

The Breath Cycle

During a breath cycle, we do two very distinct things that create very different feelings. We inhale and we exhale and they don't feel the same.

Breathing in makes me feel more up, more lifted and almost lighter. And it also creates this growing feeling, like we are expanding, which we literally are.

Breathing out makes me feel more grounded, more downwards. It is also a shrinking or contracting feeling and at the same time it makes me feel heavier in a way.

So, inhalation and exhalation create different feelings and can be used in different ways when we dance, to express these different feelings in the music.

When we breathe in, we can connect it to softer, more airy moves that give an expanding feeling. I think it makes sense to connect it to a high or rising pitch since breathing in gives this "up" feeling.

Breathing out can be connected to heavier and contracting moves. And regarding the pitch, breathing out makes more sense to a pitch that is low or going down.

We can use the breathing to highlight these feelings of direction, up or down, as well as expansion or contraction breathing in and out. We can use it for soft and airy sounds, or for grounded and heavy sounds.

Ways of Breathing

Breathing can also be very different depending on how we do it:

- First of all, is the breath the only thing we do to the music? Or do we use the breath together with a move to highlight something in the music?
- Secondly, do we do it fast, to accent something fast, or do we do it slow, to accent a slower and more extended sound or move?
- Third, do we do it more staccato, to highlight something played staccato or do we want to give it more of a legato feeling?
- And lastly, do we do it in one breath, or do we do it in several divided and shorter ones?

We can breathe in many different ways, and it can many times be matched to the music. And when we also match it to our partner, we create that extra layer of connection.

Sometimes it still impresses me how easy it is to make someone catch on to and follow my breath. It can be enough to stand in front of them, without any physical contact and just breathe to make them start breathing in sync. It is not even necessary to have a chest connection to feel our partners breathing and pick up on it.

Important to remember though is that in couple dancing, highlighting sounds with our breath makes the most sense when our partner can pick up on it. When we are very separated and move more around it is more difficult.

And, even more importantly, we cannot do it all the time. The first priority for our breathing is to keep a steady flow of oxygen to the brain and our muscles. Overusing our breathing for musicality might make us look too robotic, and we might forget to take advantage of other opportunities to play with the music. But sometimes the breath can be a nice way to play with the music.

Exercises

Perception

- ‣ Listen to some music from your dance genre and listen for sounds that seem expanding or contracting. If there are none, see if you can find places where the pitch is rising for several notes in a row, or falling for several notes in a row. What could you do with your breath to these sounds or passages?

Expression

- Listen to some music from your dance genre and try breathing to the music when you dance – for four beats you inhale with your nose, and the next four you exhale. Think only of the breathing. If your music is very fast, with a very high BPM, try inhaling for eight beats and then exhaling for eight.

- The Ninth Skill -
Putting it All Together

So, we can move to the beat, play with different tempos, dance in accordance to the dominant feeling of the song, and also use the different sonic attributes of sounds to express the music better. We can use the silence in the music, predict and prepare for what is going to happen and we can also play with the vocals and different actions in the music. We can even use our breathing to express the music in the best way possible.

Returning to our translation metaphor, this is the complete translation, getting everything in there. The right pronunciation, the intonation, the right tonality, and more. There is just one difference. I think a translation can be objectively better or worse. Dance is different. Dance is art.

There can be many different interpretations. And there is also one big problem.

We cannot express every sound we hear according to its sonic attributes at the same time as we dance on the beat, use the base with different timing and dance on the syncopations while finding the dominant feeling and expressing the silences at the same time as we play with words and breathe together with our partner, while constantly predicting and preparing for what is going to happen in the music.

Just reading that makes me feel exhausted. We would look like we have some kind of seizure if we tried. It would also be quite overwhelming for someone watching it. There would be too much happening to be able to take in.

And, to be honest I seriously doubt it is even possible to express the dominant feeling of a song at the same time as we do all these other things. I think it would actually be impossible to do it all at the same time.

Making Choices

Since we can't do it all, we have to make some choices. All the separate skills of musicality we talked about in this book are examples of musicality in themselves. But making this choice of what exactly to dance to is the real art of musicality.

The ninth and last skill is about making those choices and putting it all together as a whole. Since we can't dance to everything all the time, we need to simply accept that fact and instead focus on what is most important. We can be aware of what is happening in the music and still choose *not* to dance to it. We choose just one or two things that we want to highlight, even if we are able to perceive much more.

It is like going to a restaurant and checking the menu. We have all these different choices, but we don't pick all of them. During a nice dinner, we might pick one appetizer, one main dish and later on a dessert. We have choices for everything, but we just pick one. Or if we have a sweet tooth, we might get two desserts.

How to Put it all Together

During the intro of a song, during the outro and also during breaks in the music there are often very few or at least fewer instruments playing. Here, the choice of what we dance to might be easier. But for the rest of the song, there will be many things "happening" all pretty much at the same time. There will be several instruments playing, several different pitches sounding, different volumes of these sounds, and different durations for each sound. This is why it is a bit difficult. We have to make that choice, all the time picking which sound or sounds we want to highlight and how we express them as dance.

How can we make these choices? Well, this is the really difficult skill in musicality. And it comes down quite a lot to feeling.

On a higher level, what does this song tell us to do? What feeling is it that we want to show in this song? How do we want our dance to be perceived? Do we want to be very expressive, or a bit more subtle?

And on a lower level, of all the elements we could express in the music, of all those sounds, which is the most interesting to express right now?

Like I said, there is a lot of feeling included in this choice, but if I say "just feel it" it might not be very helpful. Here are some things I see influencing this choice.

Musical aspects

Volume

In a song, the volume of different sounds is one component that will influence what part of the music we choose to dance to, what instrument we choose to highlight in that specific moment. If an instrument has a high volume it will usually be more likely that we dance to it. Because the louder a specific sound, the more attention it asks for from the dancer.

We talked about whispering and shouting before. So it makes sense to dance to louder sounds. And maybe at first we would pay more attention to someone shouting. But someone whispering might also have something interesting to say. It can be the same with music. The louder sounds might call for a lot of attention. They might be the obvious choice. But the quiet sounds might tell an equally interesting story. What we choose to dance to will be influenced by this, but ultimately it is a personal choice, depending on how we hear the music and how we want to be perceived as dancers.

Competition

The fewer different sounds we hear, the less competition an individual sound has, and the more likely we are to dance to it. The more instruments playing, the more competition, the more we have to choose from, and the less likely we are to dance to a specific instrument.

And even if an instrument is playing at a low volume, if it is the only instrument playing, or one of few, the low competition will still make it quite likely that we dance to it.

Novelty

Just like the volume can influence what calls for our attention in a song, a sound that is "new" and hasn't played before can also call attention to itself. Since we are the physical representation of the music it makes sense to show it in our dance when something new happens in the music.

So, the newer a sound is in a song, the more it makes sense to dance to it. In the same way, if it is not new, it might not make that much sense to start dancing to it long after it started playing, unless it all of a sudden calls for attention for other reasons.

When we start dancing on something and it keeps repeating over and over it will become less interesting to highlight. The novelty wears off. It might become too repetitive to dance to, even if it is pretty dominant. Doing the same move to the same sound or sounds over and over can be like telling the same joke 10 times. It might be funny the first two times, but then it gets kind of boring. So, we might start highlighting it, but sooner or later it is not interesting anymore.

Appearance

If novelty is about how new something is. The appearance is about how something enters the music. An instrument can enter all of a sudden, or it can appear slowly, growing in volume. If an instrument enters very slowly, maybe the moment never comes when we really notice the change. Maybe that increase in volume is so slow that it never really feels like a real change in the music. It is just "there". But when we realize this it might not make as much sense to start dancing to it, since it has been playing for quite some time already.

On the other hand, it makes total sense to dance to instruments that make a fast entry, that appear all of a sudden. Then we show in our dance that we noticed the change in the music. When a new instrument or sound enters fast enough, it gives us reason to highlight it in our dance.

Distinctness

This is about how distinct or how different a sound is. It can be distinct compared to other instruments playing, and maybe also for that specific genre of music. A very distinct sound asks for a lot of attention. And then it would probably make sense to express it in our dance. Otherwise it would seem as if we didn't hear it. The more distinct a sound, the more attention it asks for and the more likely we are to dance to it.

Predictability

Of course, if we could never predict a sound, if it would come as a total surprise, we couldn't do much with it. The more unpredictable a sound is, the less we can use it in our dance. If it is truly impossible to predict we could only catch it if we already knew the song.

We have already talked about prediction and preparation, and we are much more likely to dance to sounds that are expected. At least the first time they appear.

We always have the possibility to express them if we know the song. And because of the repetition, we have a chance to catch that sound also when it comes back, when the music repeats itself.

But everything else equal, the more unpredictable a sound, the more difficult it is to catch it, and the less likely we are to dance to it. But on the other hand, the more interesting it becomes to actually catch it.

Conclusion

If we try to conclude this part about musical aspects, normally we will be more likely to use a specific sound if:

- It has high volume
- It has little competition
- It is new
- It appears suddenly
- It is distinct
- It is easy to predict

Special note about accents

One special ingredient in music often lives up to all of the above - the accents. First of all because they often have a high volume. Other instruments might also stop playing, or play at a lower volume during the accent, so there is less competition. The accents are also something that is "new" in the music, they appear suddenly and are often also quite distinct.

Taking all this into account, it makes total sense to do something with an accent when it first appears. And if it makes total sense to do something, and the dancer does nothing with it, it can look a bit weird. In couple dancing the follower might wonder if the leader is hearing the same music. Many accents are so obvious that it seems like we are not listening to the music at all if we do nothing.

An accent can sometimes be hard to predict when it comes the first time. And of course, this makes it difficult to express. We might miss it the first time. But then we could at least try to catch it the second time it comes, if it is something we can express with our bodies. Thanks to the repetition in music, it is likely it will come again.

Dancer aspects

The musical aspects are part of putting it all together. The other part is the dancer aspects. This covers both how good we are as dancers, but also what we personally listen to more in the music and how we want to be perceived as dancers.

Meaningfulness

How well we are able to express a sound depends on our dance skills and musicality. The more difficult a sound is to catch and express, the fewer dancers will probably try to express it. Only the really skilled dancers will be able to catch any type of sound.

To be able to express a sound there are some different hurdles we need to pass:

- Firstly, our ability to perceive music might not be very good enough yet. In that case we might not even notice, and much less pay attention to, some specific sounds.
- Secondly, maybe we would notice a sound, but not be creative enough to know how we could express it in any way that makes sense.
- Thirdly, maybe our dance skills are not good enough. We have the creativity. We can imagine what to do, but we simply can't do it.
- And lastly, in the case of couple dancing, we might believe our partner can't express the sound we want to express.

In all these cases, it is not very meaningful to even try. If we can't even perceive the sound, lack the creativity or the dance skills it will not make sense to try. And when we dance couple dances, we also have to take our partner's level into account. If a partner isn't able to follow what we want to express, it will not be meaningful to try it.

We will need some kind of common understanding. We need to find more or less the same level of understanding in the language we are speaking. The follower needs to interpret the signals right. It is not enough to send the signal if it is not understood, or if the follower can't respond to it right.

Of course, we can never know for sure if our partner can express the music the way we want to. But often it is possible to get a good idea of what they can do pretty fast. We can start slow and easy, and from there keep building up, raising the level.

Some of the musicality skills we have talked about are relatively easy to both lead and to follow. Others, like some of the aspects of sounds, can be more difficult. And for some of them, like articulation, it is not absolutely necessary that both partners articulate the move in exactly the same way, as long as both of them do it with the right timing.

In couple dancing, we always have to adapt to the level of our partner. We can choose to challenge their level a bit, but we should make sure to pick a level that makes it into a comfortable and enjoyable dance. Leading and following have to be meaningful. Dance has to be meaningful. If it is not, we have to avoid using that sound in our dance. We need to choose what to dance to so that it makes sense and is possible to handle also for our partner.

Continuity

Let's say we have started using slow moves on the base in a song. If the feeling of the song doesn't change, it makes quite a lot of sense to keep using slow moves on the base. Not all the time maybe, because we want to have some variation. But since all music is built on repetition, it makes a lot of sense to keep some repetition in the dance. The idea of continuity in the dance is to create a home, somewhere we can relax a bit. We know what to expect in terms of what we dance to and what kind of moves we do. It makes the dance a bit more predictable.

The dominant feeling of the song will affect the dominant feeling of our dance. And the dominant feeling of our dance is what creates this continuity.

Quite often when we dance, the most common tempo we use is on tempo. It adds to this feeling of a safe home, and it can be ok to dance mostly on tempo for many songs. If the song feels a bit slower, we often dance on tempo with some slower moves on half tempo in each count of eight. And if it is faster, we mostly dance on tempo and add some moves on double tempo. This is part of finding the dominant feeling, and when we make this choice for a song and mostly stick to it, we keep the continuity.

Another aspect of continuity is to use the same elements in the music in similar ways. So, if the music is offering a call and response between two different instruments, for example, we might use the same type of moves for that call and response also the second time it appears. This creates comfort and familiarity and keeps the continuity. But we might not want to be super predictable all the time. We might want to change it up sometimes.

Interruption

We have already talked about it before, all music is built on repetition and variation. Just like the musician is using some variation in the music, most more advanced dancers also use variation in their dance and what they choose to dance to. Repetition gives us some continuity, and the variation gives us the possibility to interrupt this continuity.

We usually try to follow the music. But some music can be very relaxed and for dance it can sometimes sound too much the same. It has too much repetition and can become, dare I say it, almost boring.

Even if it is comfortable and safe, we don't want to stay at home all the time. Sometimes we want to go on vacation and see something new. We want to change the scenery. Go on a road trip. Maybe a little adventure.

If we want to get more variation in our dance, we can introduce our own interruption, even if the music didn't change much.

If we have been dancing slow for some time, maybe we want to speed up a little bit? Or if we have been choosing faster moves maybe we want to slow down? As long as we don't totally break the feeling in the music.

When we make this choice, it can help to think if there is anything in the music that has changed to this upcoming step. Even if the feeling is the same, is there something in the music that says we could change the tempo? Could we use the change in pitch of an instrument to move up or down, in a vertical plane? Could we take a bigger or smaller step than just before? What does the timbre tell us? Does it sound dramatic?

We want to create a full picture, a more balanced dance, varying more between different tempos, different dynamics, and different aspects of sounds. The dominant feeling is there, providing a safe home, and continuity makes it easy to recognize it and follow it in the dance. And then we interrupt this sometimes. We go on a little road trip. We try to create a more interesting experience, balancing the continuity with some interruption, catching the variation in the music, and sometimes changing what we dance to to create an interruption of our own. As long as we don't totally break the feeling.

Personal Expression

Musicality is very much about personal expression. As mentioned, I believe there are some ways to interpret the music that makes more sense than others.

I believe most of the skills we have talked about so far can be done in a more "right" way, even if musicality is not science. Moving on the beat, as opposed to off the beat. A sound with a long duration fits with a move that is slower and longer duration. A sound with some vibrato might need a move with some vibrato to really be described well. And if we flip it around, dancing on double tempo when there is nothing in the music with this tempo doesn't make sense.

So, I believe all the previous skills we have talked about can be done more or less "right". But we can't do them all right at the same time. It is when we put this all together that the personal expression really comes into play. It is when we pick and choose what exactly to use in the music that we add our personal touch. What we express in our dance is highly personal.

First of all, our dance will usually be very influenced by the way we perceive the music. If we have a tendency to listen more to the rhythm, we will usually express it more in our dancing. And if we listen more to the melody, we will use that instead.

Our personal expression will also depend on how we are as a person. Are we a bit more introverted, maybe less expressive in general? Then our dance might also be a bit like that. Or are we very extrovert and expressive?

It can also be influenced by how we want to be perceived by the audience or our dance partner? Do we want to be very romantic or maybe very funny on the dance floor? Maybe we want to be a very expressive dancer, making big and bold moves, even if we are introvert? Or maybe we want to be more subtle, dancing on the small details? Even if there are sounds that dominate in volume, we might choose to express some more subtle sounds if we want our dance to be more subtle.

Maybe we want to be a stable and reliable dancer, one that has a lot of continuity and is easy and relaxing to dance with? Or maybe we want to be more creative, a bit unpredictable, interrupting the continuity with different and unexpected interpretations of the music, constantly surprising our partner?

Conclusion

If we try to conclude this part about dancer aspects, normally we will try to:

- Dance to what is meaningful to us and our partner.
- Find our own balance between continuity and interruption.
- Use our own personal expression, both how we personally hear the music, and also how we wish to be perceived.

There are many different aspects to this. Personal expression is what ultimately puts it all together. It takes all the ingredients we have been talking about in this book and mixes them up following our own recipe so that we give our dance its personal flavour. It takes our level of dancing into account, our partners level if we have one, it makes a decision on all things happening in the music and picks what to dance to. It strikes the balance between continuity and interruption. And it takes into account both how we are as a person and how we want to be perceived.

There is constantly a choice to be made. Both on what to do, and on how to do it. When we talk about textures, for example, we really want to get the feeling right. We should not be too subtle, but we also cannot exaggerate if we want to represent the music in the best way possible.

Some of these aspects of sounds are easier to evaluate objectively. When we do a move, we need to adapt it to the volume for example. If it is loud in the music, it makes sense to make it loud in our dance. If the duration is long in the music, it makes sense to make the duration long in our dance.

Other aspects are more difficult, or open for interpretation. They can be more subjective. How soft is a sound? What is an "airy" sound? What does the timbre actually tell me, on a detailed level, on how to do a move? How much is "a lot of energy"?

These aspects that are more open to interpretation will all be expressed, heavily influenced by our own personal expression.

Ultimately, the personal expression is what gives us the freedom to express ourselves as we wish. It always comes down to this. Dance is art. It is subjective. We hear the music in different ways, and therefore we will also express the music in different ways when we dance.

Exercises

Perception

- Listen to some music from your dance genre. Pick one single instrument and listen to it - how can we dance to it? Think about the durations so you can play with different tempos. Think about the other aspects of sounds, so you can catch the different textures and the pitch for example. Then pick another instrument from the same song. Repeat for as many instruments as you like.

Expression

- Listen to some music from your dance genre. Pay attention to it and try to "paint" the music with only your hands and arms. If you are dancing with a partner, put the palms of your hands together in front of you and let one of you "paint" the music. The other one just follows the hands and "listens". Think about the size of moves, the tempo, the textures, everything we have talked about. Then change who is the painter. Repeat for as many songs as you wish.

FINAL WORDS

I think the absolute best way to become a better dancer is to take good classes and then dance a lot, sometimes with deliberate practice and sometimes with hours and hours on the dance floor. And I think the absolute best way to improve our musicality is to listen to a lot of music, try to focus on different aspects of the music, both when dancing, and at other times when we are just listening. And then think about how the skills in this book could be used to express that music with the body.

Just like we need to practice a move until it is in muscle memory, we need to get to the point where we feel the music like in "muscle memory". When we can feel the music like in muscle memory then it becomes really enjoyable to dance and play with the music. It will come to us naturally, without thinking about exactly what we are doing and why.

Musicality is Personal

In this book we have gone through a lot of different aspects of musicality. I believe there are some things that make more sense than others. I believe there is a dominant feeling in most music. I believe it makes more sense to express specific sonic attributes in certain ways. Different textures catch this. All the first eight skills in musicality cover this.

With this being said, I do think that musicality exists in many different forms. There is no objectively right way to interpret music in dance. Rather, there are many subjectively right ways of interpreting music. We all hear music slightly differently. We will all express it slightly differently in dance. And this is where the last skill, putting it all together, comes in.

There is so much going on all the time. Music has so many different qualities. And the more going on, the more difficult it can be. The more there is to choose from. Exactly what qualities one specific dancer hears, chooses to pay attention to and expresses in their dance might not be the same as what someone else chooses.

As a solo dancer, we can choose to express ourselves exactly as we wish. But in couple dancing, sometimes we need to adapt. First of all, we need to adapt to the level of our partner. We might also need to adapt a bit to how he or she hears the music. It will be easier to lead when we do. And when we find a partner that hears the music the same way, or at least very similar, it is like magic. Everything we do becomes easier. The leader hears the music in a certain way, and the follower is already prepared to do a certain type of movement because they hear the music the same way. If there is a faster part coming up, both bodies will be a bit tenser already. They both engage their cores and prepare to do something fast. Or they might both relax a bit more to do something slow, if it is something that requires more flexibility.

We all have our own personal way of hearing the music. When we dance together, the magic really happens when we find the common ground and hear the music the same way.

Musicality is Natural

Musicality is also natural and relaxed. It is not analytical or forced. In this book, I have covered many different aspects of musicality and some tips on how we can use them. I have tried to break it down and explain it as well as I can. If we want to figure out what musicality is, I think that it is necessary to go into this kind of detail and almost make it too analytical.

But the idea is not that we should fill our brains with all this and then go to the dance floor and execute it, dance as if we were some kind of musicality factories. That way we would probably make it far too mechanical and robotic. The idea is to be aware of what is happening and make a choice. We need to feel more, and it needs to come more naturally. So, when we dance to enjoy, we need to get back up on a higher level. Leave it more to our feelings, let it come to us.

To get to that level we need to practice a lot, but practice a little at a time. Take it step by step. We can practice each skill pretty focused. We can go down to this detailed level from time to time, and really think about what we do. But we shouldn't think about everything. And we shouldn't think about it all the time. Only some of the things, some of the time when we practice. This attempt at making an analytical breakdown of musicality is to offer some help on the way, some new ideas on how to listen to the music, what we could do with it, and to have some concrete things we can practice.

We can't count the steps on the floor all the time. We can't think all the time. In the beginning, it is ok. When we practice something, it is ok. But we also need to turn off our brain a bit and just feel. Once we are on the social floor we need to be relaxed.

If we think too much, we will lose the natural connection between our dance and the music. It must come naturally, and it will, if we listen to a lot of music and dance a lot. The more we dance, the easier it will become to find that feeling. And the less we will need to think.

The music is a language. Our job is to interpret that language and translate it into dance. So, let's go bring it alive!

But first, don't miss to turn the page for the five last tips!

FIVE TIPS TO IMPROVE MUSICALITY

Here are some more general suggestions on how to improve musicality:

- Listen to a lot of music. Really try to understand it. Sometimes it can be playing in the background while you are doing something else, like a passive musicality training. And sometimes you can listen actively, thinking about the different skills we have covered in this book. Try to listen to as many different genres of music as possible.

- Take musicality classes. Search out some classes with really good teachers. Sometimes you can even try to go to musicality classes for dances that are not your preferred dance style. You will learn a lot, and maybe see things from a different perspective.

- Watch other people dance. When you watch other people dance you see them move in different ways than you do. You will notice new things in the music, things that they hear and pay attention to but that you might not. You will also see how they express it in a different way than you do, with different moves, textures and a different feeling. It will open your mind to a different musicality, expand it and it will make your own musicality richer when you start hearing those things as well.

- Dance a lot. Dance on your own. And if you are a couple dancer, dance also with a partner. Actually, as many different partners as you can. Really try to focus on different musicality skills from time to time. And at other times, just relax and let your musicality come naturally.

- Go to www.musicalitycourse.com and sign up for the course. There we will go through more than 60 different exercises to improve your musicality, covering all the different musicality skills.

Thank you so much for reading this book. It will make me very happy if it helps you with your musicality and dancing in some way. Feel free to tell others about it, and feel free to tell me what it has done for you, or how I can improve it in possible future revisions. Just send me an email at: kristoferbookings@gmail.com.

Good luck and I will see you on the dance floor!

CONNECT WITH ME

Feel free to connect with me. For whatever reason—if there is something you think I should add to the book or something that could be explained better, if you want to book me for classes, or some other collaboration.

kristoferbookings@gmail.com

Also feel free to connect with on my primary social media profiles. I would be happy to see you there:

facebook.com/kristofermencakdancer
youtube.com/@kristofermencak
instagram.com/kizombaflow
tiktok.com/kristofermencak

Please leave a review of this book on Amazon, especially if you like it! And feel free to tell friends about it! It would be much appreciated.

See you on the dance floor!

Kristofer

OTHER BOOKS BY KRISTOFER MENCÁK

In the Dance Series

"The Secrets of Social Dance – How to Become a Popular Dancer", on Amazon.com.

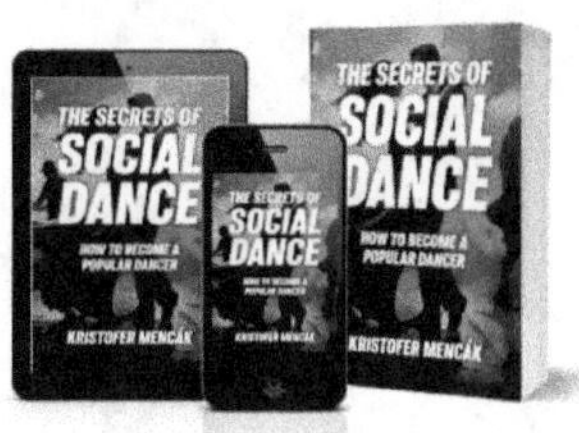

Other

"Unsuck Life – The Tips Tools & Tricks for How to Change What Sucks and Improve What Doesn't", on Amazon.com.

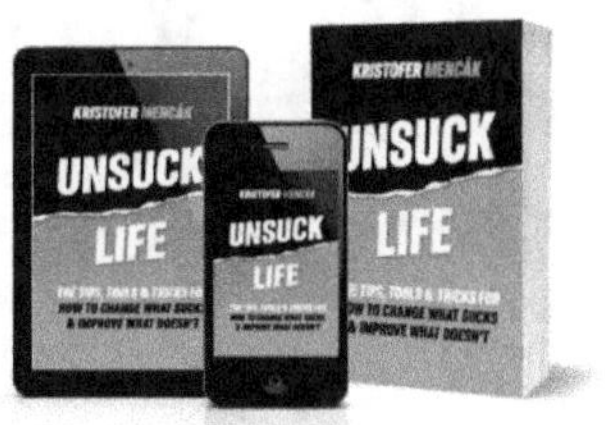